# THE FUTURE OF BIOETHICS ⁛

# The Future of Bioethics ::

Howard Brody

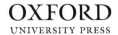

OXFORD
UNIVERSITY PRESS

2009

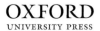

# OXFORD
UNIVERSITY PRESS

Oxford University Press, Inc., publishes works that further
Oxford University's objective of excellence
in research, scholarship, and education.

Oxford New York
Auckland Cape Town Dar es Salaam Hong Kong Karachi
Kuala Lumpur Madrid Melbourne Mexico City Nairobi
New Delhi Shanghai Taipei Toronto

With offices in
Argentina Austria Brazil Chile Czech Republic France Greece
Guatemala Hungary Italy Japan Poland Portugal Singapore
South Korea Switzerland Thailand Turkey Ukraine Vietnam

Copyright © 2009 by Oxford University Press, Inc.

Published by Oxford University Press, Inc.
198 Madison Avenue, New York, New York 10016
www.oup.com

Oxford is a registered trademark of Oxford University Press.

Library of Congress Cataloging-in-Publication Data
Brody, Howard.
The future of bioethics / Howard Brody.
   p. ; cm.
Includes bibliographical references and index.
ISBN 978-0-19-537794-1
1. Bioethics.   2. Medical ethics.   I. Title.
[DNLM:   1. Bioethics.   WB 60 B8645f 2009]
QH332.B76 2009
174'.957—dc22
2008024355

9 8 7 6 5 4 3
Printed in the United States of America
on acid-free paper

# ACKNOWLEDGMENTS ⊞

The contents of this book took shape when, for the first time in a quarter-century, I put myself on the bioethics job market, and came to realize that I had gotten out of the habit of asking a basic question—where ought the field of bioethics go in the future? I developed the next version in the process of assembling a graduate seminar called "The Future of Bioethics" upon taking up my new post as director of the Institute for the Medical Humanities at the University of Texas Medical Branch at Galveston. I am grateful to all the administrators and faculty of UTMB who did so much to make me feel welcome and to ease my transition. The students who attended my seminar helped greatly by assembling detailed bibliographies and recording class discussion notes and summaries. I must therefore give special credit to my students: Karin Ewer, John "Paulie" Gaido, Daniel Goldberg, Randall Horton, Julie Kutac, Krisann Muskievicz, and Nobue Urushihara Urvil. I was also greatly assisted by the highly professional and accommodating staff of the Institute, especially my own administrative assistant, Beverly Claussen, and Donna Vickers, administrative coordinator of the graduate program.

At this stage I had a list of issues that I thought needed to be addressed in any future bioethics worthy of the name; but I still lacked a sense of their cohesion. Criticisms of presentations by my colleagues in the Institute for the Medical Humanities, and by editor Peter Ohlin and the readers for Oxford University Press, took me to the present stage of writing. The interdisciplinary breadth of comments and criticisms that I received from my Institute colleagues certainly reinforced my views that bioethics, to be properly practiced, requires a strong and rigorous interdisciplinary base (Chapter 2). I have tried in the chapter endnotes to credit each individual from whom I have taken specific ideas or suggestions, and I apologize to those whom I have no doubt passed over accidentally.

During the final stages of editing, I had the good fortune to work especially with Lynda Crawford of Oxford University Press and Aloysius Raj of Newgen Imaging Systems. I am grateful to both of them for their patience and attention to detail.

# CONTENTS ⁙

# THE FUTURE OF BIOETHICS ⁛

# 1 ::

# Introduction

*"Is there any point to which you would wish to draw my attention?"*
*"To the curious incident of the dog in the night-time."*
*"The dog did nothing in the night-time."*
*"That was the curious incident," remarked Sherlock Holmes.*[1]

I became involved in the field of bioethics in June, 1972, when I attended the first National Conference on Teaching Medical Ethics, sponsored by the Hastings Center, in Tarrytown, New York.[2] After I had served my apprenticeship (completing medical school and a residency in family medicine, and graduate work in philosophy), I set out to establish a career as a teacher and practitioner of bioethics in an academic setting. I became particularly interested in bioethics' nocturnal canines—the issues that were making no commotion and so not receiving the attention that they deserved. This tendency led me to address the role of narrative in medicine and in bioethics,[3] to consider issues of power,[4] to explore some concerns at the interface between professional ethics and health policy,[5] and finally to delve a bit into the history of medical ethics.[6]

In the fall of 2005, after a very satisfying quarter-century at the Center for Ethics and Humanities in the Life Sciences at Michigan State University, I considered moving to the Institute for the Medical Humanities at the University of Texas Medical Branch (UTMB) in Galveston. I was asked to propose the obligatory "vision statement" for assuming the directorship of the Institute. I was thus led to explore, more systematically than I had for some years, what might be missing in today's bioethics scholarship and practice, and how these missing elements might better be attended to.

The inquiry passed through several stages. At first, I had a disconnected laundry list of various bioethics topics.[7] I could give, I thought, a reasonable account of how bioethics might be improved and expanded if it paid more attention to this or that particular dog; but I could not discern any family resemblance among the chihuahuas and Great Danes that I had assembled. Finally, what seemed to crystallize the process for me was the realization that I was working on a sort of sequel to my earlier book, *The Healer's Power*. Each chapter, in its own way, was trying to answer a question of this sort: Is bioethics succeeding in speaking truth to power? Is bioethics effectively taking the side of the relatively less powerful, or siding with those who would exploit them?

This reformulated concept of the project led to the following list of topics that needed to be addressed:

- Bioethics' Interdisciplinary Base
- Patient-Centered Care
- Evidence-Based Medicine and Pay-for-Performance
- Community Dialogue
- Cross-Cultural Concerns
- Race and Health Disparities
- Disabilities
- Environmental and Global Issues
- Critical Assessment of New Technologies

In this chapter I will deal with a number of preliminary tasks. I will see what sort of definition of "bioethics" is needed for us to move forward. I will briefly ask what evidence there is that the list of topics I propose is genuinely being neglected at present within the field. I will spend a good deal of space explaining why a number of apparently likely topics were not placed on the list. Finally, I will explain the ordering of the remaining chapters.

## ⠃ What, Exactly, Is Bioethics?

Many bioethicists, myself included, have approached the field via training in philosophy. Philosophers learn that the proper way to begin any inquiry is to define one's terms. I would, therefore, appear remiss for having proceeded this far without having defined "bioethics." My intent, actually, is to try as hard as I can not to offer any such definition. I must therefore give some account of myself.

My intended audience for this book consists primarily of those already committed to, or at least interested in, this thing we call bioethics. I want to contribute to the ongoing conversation among us as to where the field is going and ought to go.[8] I believe that I have some fresh and interesting things to say; and I believe that those who have been attending to the ongoing conversation of the field will readily recognize the relevance of what I will have to offer. As long as that happens, we are all operating with a rough, implicit definition of the thing we call bioethics. Until we find ourselves at cross purposes, in a way that a more precise definition will help resolve, I see no reason to stop to develop a formal definition.

If pressed to say more, I would fall back on Judy Andre's very promising approach to bioethics as *practice*.[9] Andre was also trained in philosophy. She came to wonder what, of all those things she learned in philosophy graduate school, she actually uses today in her work, and what things that she needs for her work did she learn elsewhere. It is tempting for philosophers to imagine bioethics as a large bookshelf, holding all the major textbooks and monographs as well as all the journals devoted to bioethics. The sum of all the information contained on that bookshelf comprises the "field" of bioethics. Andre rejects that static view, and believes that bioethics is not a body of information, but a practice, "a coherent, complex set of activities, with its own distinctive goals and standards of excellence."[10] Accordingly she begins her book by describing what she actually did during one week of her professional life. I will assume that most practitioners of bioethics could provide a similar catalogue of activities. The list would include varying proportions of:

- teaching audiences ranging from university undergraduates to medical students, residents, and practicing health professionals;
- serving on clinical or research ethics committees and conducting consultations on ethical issues in clinical settings;
- conducting research and writing up the results for publication, again in a variety of venues ranging from academic peer-reviewed journals to local newspapers and hospital bulletins.[11]

Other activities would also appear on this list, based on the local setting and that particular individual's interest and training.

Andre characterizes the "goals that define bioethics" as "[k]eeping moral space open, providing language and skills within it, identifying moral problems and helping create solutions for them."[12] The domain within which bioethics pursues these goals is generally that of health care, health professions education, health policy, and biomedical research. Bioethics pursues its goals within its domain in a way that Andre characterizes as someplace in between pure scholarship and political activism. Bioethics, she believes, tries to change the world by stimulating "moral development within ourselves and others, a development that comprises moral perception, reflection, and action."[13]

Daniel Callahan agrees with Andre that bioethics can be viewed as a practice, but questions whether it is as unified as she claims. He instead offers a typology of five bioethics "practices":

- clinical bioethics
- foundational bioethics
- regulatory bioethics
- cultural bioethics
- health-policy bioethics

Of these, my major focus in this volume will be "foundational bioethics," with a degree of "cultural bioethics" thrown in. Since my philosophical approach will be pragmatic rather than foundational or essentialist, I dispute the term "foundational."[14] But my major focus will nevertheless be on bioethics as an intellectual pursuit. I will be addressing the intellectual problems bioethics undertakes to address, and the intellectual tools that it brings to the process.

It might seem that I have contradicted myself by first, approving of Andre's conception of bioethics as practice, and then apparently retreating to the model of bioethics as a shelf full of books (to which I have the nerve to try to add yet one more). I hope that by the time that I am done any apparent contradiction will have dissipated. There are various ways in which one may intellectualize. Some ways seem to prize the intellectual pursuit as an end in itself. Other ways take for granted that the intellectualizing will be of value only to the extent that it aids practical, real-world work. I hope to engage here in the latter sort.

I believe that what I have said here comprises a sufficient definition of "bioethics" for us to proceed. My goal in this conversation is to open some doors that bioethics may previously have been hesitant to look behind. I am concerned that the more we try prematurely to define "bioethics" precisely, the more likely some of those doors are to remain shut.

## ⸬ Is There Evidence?

In some presentations based on early versions of the chapters in this book, I was asked whether I had any evidence that the "neglected" areas of bioethics that I had identified were, indeed, relatively neglected.

My standard answer, after I became used to the question, was that I was content to offer a strictly subjective impression. After all, my claim was, not that these areas were receiving no attention at all, but that they received less attention *than they deserved*—and by what yardstick could I measure how much attention each deserves?

As I was nearing completion of the project, however, I received my copy of *The Oxford Handbook of Bioethics,* with a copyright date of 2007. I did a quick search of the table of contents and index, with the results shown in the following Table 1.1.

TABLE 1.1  Pages devoted to various topics, *The Oxford Handbook of Bioethics* (2007)[15]

| Topic | Number of Pages |
|---|---|
| End-of-life care | 107 |
| Genetics | 97 |
| Research ethics | 97 |
| Global/international health issues | 52 |
| Cloning and stem cells | 52 |
| Organ transplant | 29 |
| Ethics of public health | 25 |
| Feminism (regarding commodification of female reproduction, only) | 24 |
| Technology (generally) | 5 |
| Disability | 2 |
| "Ecogenetics" | 1 |

*Not listed in index:*
anthropology
community
cross-cultural
culture
environment
evidence-based
family medicine
history
interdisciplinary[16]
patient-centered care
pay-for-performance
Potter, V.R.
primary care
race
religion
sociology

I offer Table 1.1 as some level of evidence that most of the issues discussed in this volume are truly under-represented in the "mainstream" bioethics literature. The major exception appears to be global health issues, and I would contend that this degree of focus on the global scene is a relatively new development (and indeed probably reflects the efforts of the editor and publisher to make this handbook a truly international as opposed to an American volume).

## ‼ The Usual Suspects: Topics Not Included

I would imagine that the reader will immediately wonder about "the usual suspects"—bioethics topics that we have become used to associating with the future of the field. I will therefore explain why a number of topics *were not* included in this volume—why those dogs were felt to be making sufficient noise already.

The reasons for excluding these topics might clarify a key assumption of this volume. Bioethics, we assume, will continue to make advances by addressing new issues that come up in health care and in the biomedical sciences. Many of these new issues will call for the bioethical equivalent of what Thomas Kuhn famously called "normal science."[17] That is, nothing especially new by way of intellectual tools or methods will be required to make an ethical appraisal of these new developments. I consider a topic worthy of inclusion in this volume only if it promises a shift toward what Kuhn called "revolutionary science." To do justice to the topics that I list, bioethics will need to develop new intellectual approaches, or at least considerably sharpen and refine old ones. The spectrum from "normal bioethics" to "future bioethics" is a continuum, so there is a lot of room for disagreement as to whether any particular topic crosses over the "revolutionary" threshold.[18]

*Genetics and genomics.* Many bioethicists have been devoting attention to the various issues raised by advances in genomic science, especially human cloning and stem cells. To some degree, the focus on the new genetics has been an artifact of funding. While the program "Ethics, Law, and Social Impact" (ELSI) received only a tiny percentage of all the funding made available to the Human Genome Project, for several years it dominated the funding sources specifically available for bioethics research.

There are two reasons not to include genetics-genomics on our "future" list. First, and most important, I remain skeptical that any new intellectual tools will be needed to address these issues, or will emerge from the careful study of these issues. Many of today's scholars appear to be mostly unaware of the body of literature generated in the mid-to-late 1970s on many of these same questions, including human cloning and the "manufacture" of human beings. At least on superficial survey, most current arguments raised both for and against the use of any new genetic technology track very closely the arguments elaborated in that earlier set of books and articles.[19] There does not appear to be all that much new under this sun.

Another, secondary, reason is my view that bioethics ought not become a part of the American claque that applauds every "new" scientific "advance" in knee-jerk fashion—an issue I will address in more detail in Chapter 11 on new medical technologies.[20] The cable news networks appear to be fully capable of "gee-whizzing" scientific discoveries without our assistance—whether we give that assistance in the form of waving pompoms over the great benefits that will result for humankind, or by cluck-clucking about the grim possibilities that essential human values will be eroded. Given all the ink that has been spilt over these supposedly pressing matters, we would imagine that, of this writing, something that arose from the new genomics was actually working and making a real difference in health care. In hindsight we might wonder whether the more serious ethical question was not whether or not to employ these powerful new tools to change human existence, but rather the blatant politicization of the funding of scientific research that led to the mapping of the human genome. We might later explore, for instance, how quickly the leading genomic scientists in the United States changed their tune from how much would be known once we completed mapping the genome (so keep that generous funding coming our way), to how little was actually known once we completed mapping the human genome (so keep that generous funding coming our way).[21]

*End-of-life care.* Bioethics, to a large extent, cut its teeth in the 1970s on end-of-life care issues. By the turn of the twenty-first century, it seemed that if anything in bioethics was comfortably settled, it was the "core" end-of-life care matters (omitting the admittedly controversial topics such as euthanasia, assisted suicide, and medical futility). The furor over the Terri Schiavo case in 2005 was profoundly disquieting to many of us because it suggested the need to revisit a certain part, if not a large part, of that settled core. Distinguished voices in bioethics soon were claiming that a major rethinking of end-of-life care was in order.[22] The President's Council on Bioethics, approaching from a different political direction, issued a report on care for the elderly that stood much of the "settled core" on its head.[23]

We will clearly need in coming years to readdress care at the end of life, including many hallowed assumptions of yesterday's bioethics. I suggest, however, that it will be done under some of the headings on our topic list, such as community dialogue, multiculturalism, and disabilities and race/ethnicity studies. I see no need to add "end-of-life care" as a separate topic area of its own.

*Feminist bioethics.* Hilde Lindemann has argued that bioethics is gendered feminine but often tries to act masculine.[24] It is gendered feminine because it has defined itself as a sort of handmaiden to biomedicine, helping address important ethical topics but without calling into question the basic worth of the biomedical enterprise itself. It often tries to act masculine because in our culture, what is feminine receives little respect. "Hard" science, for instance, is viewed as masculine, so it is no mystery that bioethics has so fallen in love with the new genomics.

If one takes Lindemann's analysis seriously, then it would seem that bioethics today is seriously lacking in feminist critique, and that a more concerted effort to address a feminist view of and approach to bioethics is sorely needed. I agree that this critique is intellectually rich and should continue. But I also note that excellent works on feminist bioethics already sit on our bookshelves—as do promising works on such closely related topics as narrative bioethics.[25]

A field such as feminism obviously cannot be reduced to a single formula. I nonetheless boldly propose that if there is a basic message that feminism (in its most useful form) offers to bioethics, it is that we need to understand how certain facts, issues, and questions turn *invisible* to us, depending on where we happen to be placed in a hierarchy of power.[26] We of the older generation of bioethicists went to school in a day when history books were about who won or lost battles, and not about who did the laundry. If women showed up in the history books at all, it was likely to reflect how occasionally women, through a variety of strange circumstances, ended up in the vicinity of a battlefield. What is ethically telling about those history books is less that they were written that way, and more that none of us thought to question why they were written that way or to imagine that they could have been written any differently. So feminism teaches bioethics that it must "learn to see" what the dominant power structure may be actively, even if unconsciously, discounting.[27]

The feminist bioethics agenda must continue to advance, but it must also be extended towards other groups that have been on the wrong end of the power equation. I believe that the feminist agenda in bioethics has made relatively more progress, and has been accorded a bit more attention, than analogous discussions relating to people of "other" cultures, races, and ethnicities; persons with disabilities; and citizens of developing countries. Chapter 6 provides the link between the feminist model of power disparities and these other topics.

*Research ethics* An anonymous correspondent painted a bleak picture of the current state of research ethics in a letter to the *Hastings Center Report,* March–April 2006. The writer described personal experience with apparently well-respected senior scientists who demanded of their students both scientific fraud and unethical shortcuts in the enrollment of research subjects, and took reprisals against any students who complained or threatened to expose such behavior. The author also mentioned other senior scientists whose behavior was described as "scrupulous." But these "scrupulous" scientists also urged the students to knuckle under to the demands of their less-scrupulous colleagues, rather than risk a premature end to their careers by blowing the whistle on their superiors' ethical lapses.[28]

For the remainder of this discussion, I will make a possibly questionable assumption: that the practices described in this letter are sufficiently widespread to be truly worrisome, instead of a local aberration. To the best of my knowledge, we do not know for sure if this assumption is true or not; and the fact that we do not know this very important information should itself be a cause of worry. (If research ethics were doing what it was supposed to be doing, would we not have tried harder to find out?)

The implications of this anonymous letter are that the research ethics enterprise has been a marked success at one level and a signal failure at another, very important level. Research ethics has been a great success in erecting a structure of institutional protections for human (and, for that matter, animal) subjects. A great number of practices exist today within institutions engaged in research having human subjects' protection as their goal. Recently, nationally renowned academic medical centers were forced to shut down all research when it was found that subjects' protection at those centers was inadequate. A very strong message is sent by this system that human subject protection is taken very seriously in research today; and many dollars and person-hours are devoted to making this complex apparatus of protection work. In this modern environment, it is very hard to imagine how some of the research scandals of the past—Tuskegee, Willowbrook, Jewish Chronic Disease Hospital—could ever recur. And putting an end to such scandals was, after all, the driving force behind the erection of this new structure of bioethical protection in the 1970s.[29]

But one would have hoped that research ethics, as a part of bioethics, would have "worked" at another level as well. To see what this failure might consist of, imagine that a very different "whistle-blower" letter had been written to the *Hastings Center Report* in 2006.

This hypothetical letter would have come from the context of patient care, not research. This letter would have claimed that there were many physicians, in positions of respect, who urged their trainees and staff to violate routinely the most basic ethical mandates of clinical medicine. For example, they routinely failed to obtain informed consent and refused to honor clear, valid advance directives. To make the case analogous to that of the research letter, we would have to imagine that the motives for these violations were purely self-serving. Perhaps the goal was income maximization. These senior physicians wished to increase reimbursement as much as they could, and would brook no opposition from trainees with ethical qualms.

What would the rest of us think of such a letter? Would we simply shake our heads that such wickedness existed, or would we be shocked? I think we would be shocked. We would be shocked at the apparent failure of the clinical bioethics enterprise to alter the thought processes of these well-placed physicians, despite thirty years of trying hard to do so.

According to this hypothetical letter, these physicians did not engage in self-deception. We could readily understand a physician who stands to make a lot of money from doing a specific surgical procedure who then decides that this procedure is much more beneficial and less risky than an objective appraisal would have it; and who then twists patients' arms to consent to the procedure. What would be striking about this hypothetical letter is the complete lack of any need for self-deception. The physicians described were quite bold and open in their complete rejection of and contempt for the basic principles of bioethics. Bioethical principles, to them, are nothing more than minor obstacles to success. These principles mean the same thing to them as highway speed laws mean to a motorist with a radar detector. This, I submit, is what would most shock us.

So, to return to the actual letter that appeared in the *Hastings Center Report*, what seems to have been the most notable failure of the research-ethics enterprise was the failure to penetrate the minds of many—perhaps the majority—of investigators. On this account, investigators are ethical not because they have internalized a set of ethical and scientific standards, but only to the extent that the regulations force them to. As soon as the regulations open up a tiny crack for getting away with something unethical, the investigators are through that crack in a flash. And that failure, in turn (even if only partial, and even if a number of scrupulous investigators exists alongside the ethical disasters), suggests that in some important way, bioethics practitioners have for the past thirty years failed to understand the task that they set out for themselves. After all, most of us thought that we were making some sort of headway during that time, and according to this one letter, at least, we have made no headway at all. A research apprenticeship under a respected senior scientist appears to be highly likely to teach the student the opposite of good research ethics.

Now, maybe this account is far too pessimistic, and maybe more scientists actually teach good ethics by the way they run their research programs. But the charge against research ethics remains—*how would we actually know that that was the case?* To what extent have practitioners of research ethics made it their business to ask what scientists actually believe, and what they teach their graduate students and fellows in the privacy of their offices and laboratories? To what extent have bioethicists, by contrast, been content merely to look at the federal rules and at the decisions made by institutional review boards (IRBs), as if that was where the real action was?

I conclude that a good deal of work needs to be done in the area of research ethics, and that that work requires the rethinking of some of our most hallowed assumptions.[30] So it might seem especially strange that research ethics is not on my "future" topic list. Of all the omissions, this is perhaps of most concern. Yet I again suggest that the intellectual tools needed for a revised and improved view of research ethics either are already well established today, or will involve one or more of the "future" topics I have listed. For example, the vexing questions about research in developing countries surely will require that we better understand bioethics in the face of multiculturalism and globalization.

Gerald Schatz surveyed the many criticisms of the state of research ethics in the United States in 2003 and came away with two basic conclusions. First, he argued that the Belmont Report remains a sound philosophical basis for the ethics of human subjects research. Second, he insisted that Hans Jonas got it basically right in 1969 when he wrote that the essential problem of research ethics was treating the research subject as a human being of full moral worth—and not, as in the popular parlance, as a "human guinea pig."[31] I agree with Schatz on these two points. Much work is required on the *practice* of the ethics of research, but—except in those areas to be further elaborated in the following chapters—I see no basic defects in its theory.[32]

*Justice and access to health care.* I write this during the early phases of the 2008 U.S. presidential campaign. It now seems likely that health-care reform will be seriously debated by many if not most of the candidates, for the first time since the failure of the Clinton health plan in 1993–1994. During the intervening years, the number of Americans lacking health insurance has increased to nearly 45 million. This number would rise to 75 million of we counted all those who lacked health insurance for at least 6 of the preceding 24 months.[33] An Institute of Medicine report attributed 18,000 deaths annually in the United States specifically to the lack of health insurance, thereby belying the claim that those going without insurance are healthy young people who simply have no need for health care or who could easily afford it if they needed it.[34]

Even when controlling for socioeconomic differences, minority populations within the United States demonstrate worse health outcomes than the majority.[35] While the entirety of factors accounting for these differences remain a mystery, at least some of the disparity seems due to lack of access to care, or at least to the right sort of care when it is most needed.

Because of these abysmal disparities and outcomes, American health care as a whole ranks very poorly in comparison with other developed countries. According to an assessment of health system performance by the World Health Organization in 2000, the U.S. health care system overall ranked thirty-seventh, placing it between those of Costa Rica and Slovenia.[36] To achieve this low standing, the United States pays much more, in terms of GDP per capita, than any other nation. The disparities between money invested and outcome achieved is so great that even poor Britons enjoy relatively better health than wealthy Americans; and lifestyle choices can explain only a small fraction of this difference.[37] It is hard to disagree with William Phillips's conclusion that today's American health care system is designed not to provide care for the ill, but rather to provide profits for corporations.[38]

Bioethicists have written many books and articles calling this system unjust, explaining in detail what makes it unjust, and calling for meaningful, comprehensive reforms. Nonetheless, its critics have accused the bioethics movement overall of slighting this important ethical issue. We have said above that bioethics should count it a failure that it has been preaching good research ethics for about three decades and the principal audience of concern appears not to have gotten the message. Is bioethics a failure because it has failed to carry the day with its message about justice and health care reform?

It is more tempting to assign the failure to the American political system than to any movement such as bioethics, as Haynes Johnson and David Broder did in their book about the defeat of the Clinton plan.[39] This is especially so given that public opinion polls suggest repeatedly that the U.S. public agrees with the bioethicists, regarding the present system as unjust and preferring a comprehensive overhaul.

A different set of concerns about bioethics' inadequacy to address some of today's health challenges was expressed by Leslie P. Francis and her colleagues. They noted the near-total absence of cases involving infectious disease from many early textbooks of bioethics, and the inclusion of infections in later editions only in the form of HIV/AIDS. Emerging infectious diseases, either arising naturally (as in the feared avian flu pandemic) or from a bioterror plot, have moved to center stage as public health worries. Francis et al. proclaim today's bioethics to be inadequate to address these concerns. They relate this to bioethics' focus on the individual and inability to address health at the population level. They note, for instance, the dual nature of the person with an infectious disease as both victim and vector. We can no longer be content to ask whether it is in that person's best interest to offer treatment; we have to consider that a failure to treat could lead to the infection of many other individuals.[40]

One response to Francis et al. is to state simply that the ethics of public health has always been something of a poor step-cousin to "medical" ethics, just as the school of public health has traditionally been seen as less important and prestigious than the medical school. Bringing public health ethics up to its proper place within the overall bioethics enterprise would soon lay to rest any fears that we are unable or unwilling to address population-level issues.

Still, it is not clear that bioethics requires any new intellectual tools, or needs to make any major conceptual advances, to better address problems of injustice in health-care access, or concerns about populations. Three issues that we will discuss as part of the future of bioethics do, however, promise to be of considerable help. First, a better appreciation of the role of racial and ethnic matters in bioethics may assist us in grappling with the problem of health disparities. Second, we might note that, until recently, when Massachusetts and later California set out seriously to address the problem of the uninsured, the state that had made the greatest headway toward serious health reform was Oregon; and Oregon was also the home of one of the most successful early "grassroots bioethics movements" utilizing the process of community dialogue. We will later have reason to ask whether, had the "Clinton plan" not proposed a specific blueprint for reform, but rather had merely created a process of five years of nationwide town meetings on health care access, it would be viewed today as a success, and comprehensive health reform would have occurred.

Third, if we look seriously at problems of globalization, we may come to see both better ways to address the injustices within the U.S. health-care system, and also to realize that our local problems pale in comparison to international injustices. We will argue that confronting globalization seriously will require us finally to take an uncompromising stand. Bioethics, to be true to its foundations, must dedicate itself to speaking up for those who currently lack a voice, including all victims of injustice. We must respect the views of those bioethicists with a libertarian viewpoint, who would regard lacking access to health care in the United States as largely a problem of misfortune, but not injustice. That debate must continue for bioethics to be intellectually rigorous. But the larger bioethics enterprise cannot remain neutral. We must in the end side with the oppressed—just as in the early days of bioethics we sided, not with the paternalistic physician, but with the patient whose voice was being ignored.


## ⁝⁝ An Outline

Having set aside the topics that do not seem to require a sufficiently revolutionary approach, or that are already receiving adequate attention, we are now ready to deal with the topics that have been placed on the "future" list. I will next address bioethics' need for an interdisciplinary base, especially if it is to be sufficiently attuned to power disparities. Then come two chapters on issues that arise especially within primary care medical specialties—patient-centered care, evidence-based medicine, and pay-for-performance. I suggest that bioethics has neglected these important issues in part because primary care lacks power and prestige among the medical specialties. Next I take up models for community dialogue, a general method by which bioethics can help to assure that disparate voices, and not just the voices of privilege, are being heard.

Then follow four chapters devoted to issues that display a problem of power disparities roughly analogous to gender relationships as seen by feminist scholars. To introduce those four chapters, I insert first an overview chapter in which I explain how I will apply the feminist model to the other topics. Then the chapters on cross-cultural concerns, race and health disparities, disabilities, and global issues follow in sequence. A section on environmental issues accompanies the chapter on global justice. The next chapter addresses the critical assessment of new technologies, and reinforces some of the issues raised regarding international justice.

In each of these chapters, I will be trying to say two things. First, in keeping with the goal of addressing bioethics' intellectual content in a way that aids and promotes bioethics as practice, I'll be trying to point out how each topic area might enhance the future work of bioethicists. Next, I will be trying to make the case that each of these topic areas, unlike the "usual suspects" previously listed in this introduction, will help move bioethics ahead in important, intellectually novel ways, and that new conceptual tools will have to be developed in order to address that topic well. As best as I can, I will try in each chapter to address both theory and practice, and to show how these are in synchrony.[41]

The last chapter is a conclusion, which includes brief discussions of other topics that might have been placed on the "future" list but that did not seem to warrant a chapter on their own. The conclusion also focuses on the question of whether and in what way bioethics ought to be viewed as an activist pursuit.

NOTES TO THE INTRODUCTION

1. Doyle AC. *The memoirs of Sherlock Holmes*, ed. C. Roden. New York: Oxford University Press, 1993, p. 23.
2. Veatch RM, Gaylin W, Morgan C, eds. *The teaching of medical ethics.* Hastings-on-Hudson, NY: The Hastings Center, 1973.
3. Brody H. *Stories of sickness*, 2nd ed. New York: Oxford University Press, 2003.
4. Brody H. *The healer's power.* New Haven, CT: Yale University Press, 1992.

5. Brody H. *Hooked: ethics, the medical profession, and the pharmaceutical industry.* Lanham, MD: Rowman and Littlefield, 2007.

6. Brody H, Meghani Z, Greenwald K. *Michael Ryan's contributions to medical ethics.* Boston: Springer (in press).

7. When the project was at the "laundry list" stage, I took the opportunity to teach a graduate seminar called "The Future of Bioethics" at the Institute for the Medical Humanities (IMH). I am grateful to Dr. Anne Hudson Jones, director of the IMH graduate program, for assisting me in this endeavor, and to the students who enrolled: Karin Ewer, John Paul Gaido, Daniel Goldberg, Randall Horton, Julie Kutac, Krisann Muskievicz, and Nobue Urushihara Urvil. I benefitted greatly from the ensuing discussions, as well as from the detailed discussion notes and bibliographies that they prepared.

8. For a brief historical overview of American bioethics to date, see Levine C. Analyzing Pandora's box: a history of bioethics. In: Eckenwiler LA, Cohn FG, eds. *The ethics of bioethics: mapping the moral landscape.* Baltimore: Johns Hopkins University Press, 2007, pp. 3–23.

9. Andre J. *Bioethics as practice.* Chapel Hill, NC: University of North Carolina Press, 2002.

10. Andre J. *Bioethics as practice*, p. 14. The concept of "practice" here used is from MacIntyre A. *After virtue: a study in moral theory.* Notre Dame, IN: University of Notre Dame Press, 1984, pp. 181–203.

11. Ruth Faden, by contrast, draws a sharper distinction between bioethics as practice and bioethics as field of study, calling for more reflection on the implications of this distinction, especially for the training of future scholars/practitioners; Faden RR. Bioethics: a field in transition. *J Law Med Ethics* 32:276–78, 2004. I will not, in this volume, address a very important issue for the clinical practice of bioethics: the need for standards for clinical ethics consultation and for the training of consultants. See for example Rubin SB, Zoloth L. Clinical ethics and the road less taken: mapping the future by tracking the past. *J Law Med Ethics* 32:218–25, 2004.

12. Andre J. *Bioethics as practice*, p. 69.

13. Andre J. *Bioethics as practice*, p. 78. I will later (in the Conclusion, Chapter 12) return to the theme that Andre introduces, of bioethics "practice" requiring an inherently activist element.

14. Callahan defines "foundational bioethics" as "exploring the ethical basis of bioethics and its relationship to the broader field of general ethics"; Callahan D. The social sciences and the task of bioethics. *Daedalus* 128:275–94, 1999, quote on p. 279.

15. Steinbock B (ed.) *The Oxford handbook of bioethics.* New York: Oxford University Press, 2007.

16. The first five chapters, on methodology in bioethics, focus nearly exclusively on philosophical methods (except for the rule of double effect which arguably is more deeply rooted in theological ethics), with no mention of appeal to other disciplines.

17. Kuhn TS. *The structure of scientific revolutions*, 2nd ed. Chicago: University of Chicago Press, 1962.

18. For this reason, my colleague William Winslade took issue with the title "future of bioethics" at a presentation in which the graduate seminar content was discussed; he recommended that the book ought to have been titled, "Issues Receiving Too Little Attention."

19. Brody H. Ethics, technology, and the human genome project. *J Clin Ethics* 2:278–81, 1991. This analysis was in part based on Brody H. Genetic engineering: sizing up the arguments in the post–Louise Brown era. In: Teichler-Zallen D, Clements CD, eds. *Science and morality.* Lexington, MA: Lexington Books, 1982, pp. 139–53.

20. Rachels J. When philosophers shoot from the hip: a report from America. *Bioethics* 5(1):67–71, 1991.

21. Guttmacher AE, Collins FS. Genomic medicine—a primer. *N Engl J Med* 347:1512–20, 2002.

22. Murray TH, Jennings B. The quest to reform end-of-life care: rethinking assumptions and setting new directions. *Hastings Cent Rep* 35(6 suppl): S52-S57, 2005.

23. President's Council on Bioethics. *Taking care: ethical care-giving in our aging society.* Washington, DC: President's Council on Bioethics, 2005; http://www.bioethics.gov/reports/taking_care/taking_care.pdf

24. Lindemann H. Bioethics' gender. *Am J Bioethics* 6(2):W15-W19, 2006.

25. See, for example, Sherwin S. *No longer patient: feminist ethics and health care.* Philadelphia: Temple University Press, 1992; Nelson HL, ed. *Stories and their limits: narrative approaches to bioethics.* New York: Routledge, 1997; Nelson HL. *Damaged identities, narrative repair.* Ithaca, NY: Cornell University Press, 2001.

26. I am grateful to Susan Squier for the reminder of the many variants of feminism that I am excluding from consideration here, in order to focus on a single concept derived from feminist work that seems to me to be most applicable to the issues that I want to address. Professor Squier recommended to me, as a good introduction to all that was missing, Kemp S, Squires J, eds. *Feminisms* (Oxford readers). New York: Oxford University Press, 1998.

27. Andre J. Learning to see: moral growth during medical training. *J Med Ethics* 18:148–52, 1992.

28. Do researchers learn to practice misbehavior? (Anonymous letter). *Hastings Cent Rep* 36(2):4, 2006.

29. Moreno JD. Goodbye to all that: the end of moderate protectionism in human subjects research. *Hastings Cent Rep* 31(3):9–17, 2001.

30. National Bioethics Advisory Commission. *Ethical and policy issues in research involving human participants.* Washington, DC: National Bioethics Advisory Commission, 2001; http://www.bioethics.gov/reports/ past_commissions/nbac_human_part.pdf

31. Schatz GS. Are the rationale and regulatory system for protecting human subjects of biomedical and behavioral research obsolete and unworkable, or ethically important but inconvenient and inadequately enforced? *J Contemp Health Law Policy* 20:1–31, 2003. For similar points see Vanderpool HY, ed. *The ethics of research involving human*

*subjects: facing the 21st century.* Frederick, MD: University Publishing Group; 1996.

32. Franklin Miller and I have argued elsewhere that a good deal of writing on research ethics today is flawed by reliance on the concept of clinical equipoise. We claim that clinical equipoise counts as a basic theoretical mistake, blurring the important distinction between research and therapeutic medicine; Miller FG, Brody H. A critique of clinical equipoise. Therapeutic misconception in the ethics of clinical trials. *Hastings Cent Rep* 33(3):19–28, 2003. Our argument, however, is not that a new theory needs to be developed, but rather that research ethics needs to get back in touch with its old theory. Gerald Schatz makes a similar point (note 31 above).

33. Welch W. Report: 82M went uninsured. *USA Today,* June 15, 2004.

34. Institute of Medicine. *Coverage matters: insurance and health care.* Washington, DC: National Academy Press; 2001.

35. Murray CJ, Kulkarni SC, Michaud C, Tomijima N, et al. Eight Americas: investigating mortality disparities across races, counties, and race-counties in the United States. *PLoS Med* 3(9) [epub], 2006

36. World Health Organization. *The World Health Report 2000: health systems: improving performance.* Geneva: World Health Organization; 2000.

37. Banks J, Marmot M, Oldfield Z, Smith JP. Disease and disadvantage in the United States and in England. *JAMA* 295(17):2037–45, 2006.

38. Phillips WR. Questioning the future of family medicine. *Fam Med* 36:664–5, 2004.

39. Johnson H, Broder DS. *The system: the American way of politics at the breaking point.* Boston: Little, Brown, 1996.

40. Francis LP, Battin MP, Jacobson JA, Smith CB, et al. How infectious diseases got left out—and what this omission might have meant for bioethics. *Bioethics* 19:307–22, 2005.

41. I am grateful to Robert Arnold, in comments on earlier drafts, for advice on clarifying the theory–practice connection.

# 2 ⚏

# Bioethics' Interdisciplinary Base

The March–April 2006 issue of the *Hastings Center Report* contained two major articles, by Bruce Jennings and Barry Hoffmaster, respectively. Jennings addressed the care of patients with traumatic brain injury, while Hoffmaster addressed "vulnerability," especially as it applies to the elderly with disabilities and their caregivers.[1]

Jennings used as a recurring motif in his paper the poetry of Wallace Stevens, particularly "The Idea of Order at Key West." Hoffmaster developed his paper around two narratives, those of his father and his mother, both in their mid-eighties.

There was a day not too long past when the majority of bioethicists would have rejected both these papers out-of-hand. Jennings's paper might have been viewed as a literary exercise rather than "real" bioethics. Hoffmaster's discussion would have been dismissed as unacceptably subjective and anecdotal.[2]

There is another reason why the two papers might have been rejected as real bioethics. My own philosophical training was in the Anglo-American analytic mode, that most commonly taught in U.S. graduate programs during the second half of the twentieth century. I am used to reading the standard paper in bioethics and feeling a high level of confidence that I have understood what the author had to say, and that I have followed the author's line of argument.

I was strongly aware, while reading both the Jennings and the Hoffmaster papers, of the *lack* of this expected sense of certainty. I am not sure that I followed either paper totally, or that I fully grasped what each author was trying to do. In important ways the papers raised more questions and offered few answers. Considering how vexing it is to try to take good care of an elderly, disabled parent, or to deal with the myriad demands created by severe traumatic brain injury, however, uncertainty and ambiguity may capture the true nature of the issues better than any formulaic answers would.[3]

One more point struck me about the two papers. I rather doubt that either Jennings or Hoffmaster can be considered a "conservative" bioethicist, as the term has lately been applied.[4] I doubt either would endorse most of the conclusions of *Taking Care,* the report on care of the elderly that was produced by the President's Council on Bioethics, under Leon Kass's leadership, in 2005.[5] But, in important ways, each paper resonated with an important theme from the report. Each struggled to help us understand what *taking care* of a patient with traumatic brain injury, or an elderly person with disabilities, requires of us. And that is significant, given the prevalence in yesterday's bioethics of articles that were designed rather to argue that these patients, in some sense, were *not worthy* of the sort of care contemplated here— that they lacked some essential quality that translated into the moral entitlement to a considerable expenditure of resources; or that the care would produce far too little real benefit to be worthwhile. No matter what turns out to be the right answer to debates over the use of scarce medical resources, this reassessing of the balance seems a worthy enterprise.

I would argue that one of the striking things about these two papers that makes them a part of the future of bioethics, rather than yesterday's bioethics, is their *interdisciplinary* quality.[6] Jennings explicitly draws on literature, while Hoffmaster, without formal literary analysis, nevertheless employs a strongly narrative approach, which could be seen as partly grounded in literature.[7] In this chapter I will explore what the future bioethics might draw from a more interdisciplinary set of methods.[8] To use Robert Martensen's felicitous phrase, what does bioethics gain from "cross-talk" with other humanities disciplines?[9]

I will discuss bioethics' relationship to literature, history, religion, and the social sciences. This list is seriously incomplete; one could immediately add philosophy, law, economics, and policy to the list and still not have exhausted all the important possibilities.[10] Nonetheless, I will suggest that these four disciplines at least provide us with some suggestive models of how the proposed "cross-talk" works when it is most effective.

## ∷ Literature

Of the various disciplines that comprise the medical humanities, literature has perhaps today the most pressing claim to be viewed as essential to bioethics, due to the emergence of what has been called "narrative ethics."[11] Anne Hudson Jones suggests that we should distinguish between "narrative ethics" on one hand, and "narrative approaches to bioethics," or "narrative contributions to bioethics," on the other. The former, she argues, suggests a reconceptualization of the basic methods of bioethics, most notably the rejection of principlism. The latter, by contrast, treats literature as a sort of handmaiden of principlism, supplementing principlist approaches without rejecting or replacing them.[12]

Jones also distinguishes between two ways that literature can be helpful to bioethics, regardless of whether one sticks one's toe in the narrative waters (narrative approaches to bioethics) or dives in (narrative bioethics). First, the *products* of literature, the texts produced by writers, can be used as ways of better understanding the lived experiences of both patients and healthcare providers. Second, the *methods* of literary criticism can be used as ways to gain further insight into important questions in bioethics.

In the first category, narratives, whether elegantly composed by the great writers studied in literature courses, or told to caregivers by patients, provide the raw material for much medical work. Rita Charon, literary scholar and practicing internist, suggests, "What literary studies give medicine is the realization that our intimate medical relationships occur in words. Our intimacy with patients is based predominantly on *listening to what they tell us,* and our trustworthiness toward them is demonstrated in the seriousness and duty with which we listen to what they entrust to us. Yes, doctors touch patients and do rather extraordinary physical things to them, but the textuality and not the physicality defines the relation."[13]

Stories, then, abound in medicine. But what does it mean, for bioethics, to think *with* stories instead of merely thinking *about* stories?[14] I have attempted elsewhere to provide an extended, even if preliminary answer to that question.[15] For our purposes here, some summary points may suffice to show at least that the conception of a narrative bioethics deserves further study.

1. To the extent that today's neuroscience is helpful in understanding the building blocks of ethical thinking, there is strong evidence

that narrative plays a fundamental role in how we deliberate and make ethical choices.[16]

2. When an action or deliberation is analyzed after the fact, it is almost always possible to identify ethical principles according to which the action taken was right or wrong. People may then argue that without the principles, one could not determine right from wrong. But we live life forward, not backward. One may argue that we reason forward more in narrative terms than in terms of principles—that we see ourselves and those we care about as unfolding life stories, and that we decide what to do based on our assessments of what would *best* make those stories come out the way we think they should. (Developing this point further, one could claim that narratives are primary and principles secondary—that principles are a sort of ethical shorthand for collections of narratives.)

3. If we focus only on ethical decisions that arise when strangers confront strangers, it will seem that principlism is the best way to resolve ethical dilemmas. But a great part of our moral lives are lived within webs of relationships, many of them characterized by some degree of intimacy. When we move from stranger ethics to the ethics of more intimate relationships, it seems natural that narrative plays a large part in our moral thinking.[17] To the extent that health professionals wish *not* to be mere strangers to their patients, and vice versa, a narratively rich ethics is called for.

4. Most ethical choices involve alternative futures. If I travel down this path, my immediate future, and that of those most affected by my actions, will proceed in a certain way; if I choose a different path, then those futures will unfold in a different manner, and so on. In short, when we consider our moral options, we "try on" narratives and then look in the mirror, in a way roughly analogous to how we might try on a suit of clothes.[18] Narrative is the best tool we possess for vicariously living those alternative futures, enabling us to make choices among them with the best possible appreciation of what those alternatives would mean *for us*.[19]

5. As narratives are the basic building blocks of moral thought, one can refute or correct a flawed or incomplete narrative only with a better narrative. The interplay between narratives and counter-narratives is therefore a critical process for narrative bioethics.[20]

Kathryn Montgomery offers a summation:

> How human beings know what is right and, before that, how we recognize
> events and situations as morally problematic, are matters that lie deeper than
> their logical representation. Although hypothetico-deductive reasoning
> is comfortingly systematic and undoubtedly useful in dealing with moral
> quandaries, the recognition and understanding of those quandaries,
> like our knowledge of culture and its values generally, is part of a more
> discursive, practical, and narrative rationality. A good physician, like other
> reliable moral agents, grasps not just the solution to an ethical dilemma but
> the action appropriate to a morally significant situation.[21]

Montgomery goes on to quote with approval John Arras: "To paraphrase
Kant, ethics without narrative is empty."[22]

In Jones's second category, bioethics uses the methods of literary criticism, not narratives per se. Perhaps most prominent in apply-
ing literary-critical methods to the work of bioethics has been Tod
Chambers. By critically analyzing how bioethics writers construct
their case studies, he has shown compellingly that the belief that the
case study is a pre-theoretical recitation of "the facts," to which ethical theory is then applied, is far too simplistic. Rather, whatever ethical theory one adheres to guides how one constructs and formulates
"the facts of the case," resulting in a text that is effectively prepro-
grammed to support and validate the author's preferred theoretical
position.[23]

Montgomery adds here that narrative and narrative studies do
not exhaust literature's contributions to ethics. She cites as examples
Joanne Trautmann Banks, in alluding to the value of drama as a way
of representing conflict both within and between moral agents, and
Anne Hunsaker Hawkins's work on the epiphanic knowledge that can
be gained via poetry, and how it might usefully be applied to medical
practice.[24]

## :: History

In an important study of the history of medical ethics, Robert Veatch
puts forth a hypothesis about the degree to which medical ethics was
in "dialogue" with other humanities disciplines between 1760 and 1980.
He argues that, following a period of fertile exchange from about 1760
to 1800 between scholars in medical ethics and those doing more general moral philosophy, medical ethics entered a period of "disrupted

dialogue." It emerged only in the 1960s with the birth of the modern bioethics movement, when once again, humanists with a background in philosophical and religious ethics became interested and involved in the world of medicine.[25]

Veatch's own background is in ethics, and he had to depart from his disciplinary base in order to do the careful historical inquiry, including a thorough investigation of primary sources, required for his book.[26] It is therefore interesting that Veatch does not seem to have considered *history* as a discipline with which medical ethics might be or ought to be in "dialogue." For example, Veatch is quite dismissive of the ethical writing of Michael Ryan (d. 1840), an Irish physician transplanted to London who wrote a section on medical ethics for his larger work on medical jurisprudence in the 1830s.[27] Yet, according to Robert Baker and Laurence McCullough, Ryan should be credited as the first author to propose what most writers on bioethics today take for granted—that there is one coherent, single thing called "medical ethics" that existed from the time of Hippocrates and the Oath, through the works of John Gregory and Thomas Percival in the eighteenth century—and that since Ryan's time incorporated the 1847 code of ethics of the American Medical Association, and culminated most recently in the bioethics movement of today.[28] By contrast, Gregory and Percival, upon whom Ryan relied for almost his entire stock of ideas about the medical ethics of his own time, saw little relationship between what they were setting out to do and what the writer of the Hippocratic Oath had done two millennia previously. Ryan's historical hypothesis may have been well or poorly justified. But it at least seems worth mentioning that he was proposing such a hypothesis, and thus implying some sort of "cross-talk" between history and medical ethics.

Veatch's book, and Ryan's work before it, illustrate one form of cross-talk between bioethics and history. Bioethics can study its own history, and seek a better understanding of its present activities by observing their historical sources and predecessors. A second form of cross-talk occurs when bioethics addresses a specific issue or topic and engages with historians about that issue. For instance, bioethicists could address the physician's duty to treat patients suffering from a highly contagious and possibly deadly disease like severe acute respiratory syndrome (SARS) in historical isolation; or they could consult the history of physicians' responses to epidemics throughout history, most recently during the AIDS crisis of the 1980s, as a tool for understanding and framing such a duty today.[29]

*Bioethics' awareness of its own history.* There were two reasons why the first generation of bioethicists, who worked during the 1970s and 1980s, would have been largely dismissive of history as applied to their own activities. First, many of the writers on bioethics, who focused especially on the principle of respect for patient autonomy, stressed the historical discontinuity between the earlier, "Hippocratic" medical ethics and the new enterprise. To caricature the point of view of these writings, the history of medical ethics from Hippocrates through Percival and the AMA, up to the middle twentieth century, was essentially the history of physician paternalism, and the new medical ethics of the 1960s and 1970s was an entirely unprecedented activity stressing respect for patient autonomy. Ironically, given that Veatch has now joined the history brigades, his own early writing has been cited by many as a depiction of this significant historical discontinuity.[30] Since all the earlier history of medical ethics was therefore tainted with paternalism, there might seem no value in studying that history when one is doing modern bioethics. Much better to leave the old ethics on the trash heap.[31]

A closely related reason to ignore the history of the field was that, since modern bioethics sprang into being with the 1960s, it followed that all the scholars working in the field during the next couple of decades already knew all that there was to know about the history of bioethics, because they had lived and created it. They were the history. Why ask historians to expound on what they all knew already?[32]

As the years have passed, these early dismissals have given rise to a much greater willingness to explore bioethics' own history, although such inquiries still remain mostly marginal within the field.[33] Scholarly histories of recent bioethics and of bioethical inquiry have appeared, probably most significantly David Rothman's *Strangers at the Bedside.*[34] These studies ask a basic question: what had to be happening in American society and in American medicine, in the middle years of the twentieth century, to cause bioethics to emerge in the form that it took, and at the time it did? Not surprisingly, the two answers to this question offered most commonly by bioethicists themselves in the early days of the field—the problem of physician paternalism, coupled with the rapid emergence of new life-saving technologies such as organ transplants and mechanical ventilation—turn out to be very partial and limited reasons for what happened and why.

At the same time, bioethicists have developed a greater curiosity about their own medical-ethics forebears. Besides Veatch's book (and laying much of the groundwork for Veatch's inquiry), one of the most important studies to date has been Laurence McCullough's analysis of John Gregory's writings, and his claim that Gregory in an important sense invented the notion of a professional medical ethics.[35] This line of inquiry represents interdisciplinary cross-talk in an explicit way. McCullough is a philosopher who has clearly made an effort to inform himself about the intellectual and social history of the Scottish Enlightenment, in which Gregory figured. As a philosopher, McCullough can claim to have a leg up on understanding the system of ethics that Gregory was constructing, and what theoretical strands it might or might not have in common with today's bioethics. Because McCullough is quite explicit in his historical assumptions, he is open to criticism from intellectual historians such as the late Lisbeth Haakonssen, who claims that he misreads Gregory in some ways because he assumes that Gregory is trying to address twentieth-century issues rather than engaging in the real dialogue that characterized the eighteenth century.[36]

For instance, most bioethicists today, on reading Gregory or Percival, tend to focus a great deal of attention on their prescriptions for disclosing the truth to the patient facing a possibly terminal outcome. This is one of the relatively few "ethical dilemmas" that appear to bridge the world of the late eighteenth century and today's medical scene. By asking what Gregory and Percival thought about the "ethics of truth-telling," we imagine that we can measure them according to a common yardstick alongside today's bioethics. By contrast, what they might have to say about the way that surgeons, apothecaries, and physicians should interact with each other in eighteenth-century English practice appears to us utterly uninteresting and uninformative. Yet, given the priorities of their own time, it might be through studying the passages relating to the three medical orders that one would discern what Gregory and Percival were really trying to accomplish in their work, while the passages on truth-telling to the dying might by contrast be less informative. (For the reader of Percival's extensive essay on truthful disclosure, written as a sort of appendix to his *Medical Ethics,* the methods by which Percival went about consulting the works of numerous colleagues and authorities on the subject, and how he assembled what he learned from all of them, might be much more informative than his own conclusions on what one should or should not say to the patient.[37] Yet I would guess that the average modern reader skips pretty quickly over all that bibliographical material in hopes of cutting to the chase to discover the "answer.")

Despite the temptation to look at authors like Gregory and Percival through modern lenses, there seems to be a growing interest within bioethics in understanding such historical figures, and their basic approach to ethics, accurately within their own social and intellectual contexts. This seems a promising recipe for productive cross-talk between history and bioethics. Much more work needs to be done, and the fruits of the inquiry need to be brought into the center of bioethics rather than remaining a marginal preoccupation.

*Historical perspectives on bioethics issues.* As with the other humanities and social science disciplines, we must ask: What strengths or advantages would bioethics forgo, if it did *not* engage in cross-talk with history and historians? The answer to this question might well vary depending on what specific bioethics topic is considered. Are any general observations useful?

Martensen contrasts the fate of history of medicine and medical ethics/bioethics through the middle and late portions of the twentieth century.[38] At the same time that medical schools began to adopt first elective and then required courses in medical ethics, the schools proceeded to drop existing courses in history of medicine. At the same time that ethics was moving into the medical schools, history was moving out. In the early and middle twentieth century, much of the most important work on history of medicine was being written by professors in medical school departments. By the later part of the century, almost all the important work was coming out of university history departments unattached to medical schools. By moving out of medical schools, the history of medicine opened itself more to the methods then popular in departments of history, which usually stressed social-history approaches. To caricature the contrast, works in history of medicine ceased to be the biographies of the great physicians of the past, and started to become accounts of human health and illness situated within the social, cultural, and intellectual life of the times and places in which they occurred.

Too often, the earlier works in exemplary medical biography left the work of the physician-protagonist unsituated, lacking any social and cultural context. Worse, the context provided was often implicit rather than explicit, and it usually amounted to the presumed trajectory from ignorance to knowledge, the inevitable march of medical progress. What happened to sick people in a past historical period was thought to be of interest only to the extent that some physician appeared among them who could exemplify the progress of medicine. And the progress of medicine, in turn, was defined solely by what today we believe to be true.

For example, under the old regime, there would be one reason only to study bloodletting in the nineteenth century—to show how certain great physicians of the day exposed its fallacies and pointed the way to a more rational system based on modern physiology and bacteriology. To the older generation of historians, it would have made little sense to study bloodletting like Charles Rosenberg has brilliantly done. Rosenberg takes us back to the heyday of humoral medicine, when it achieved the signal triumph of being accepted unquestioningly as *the* medical system by both the educated physician and the informed lay public.[39] Ironically, humoral medicine achieved this success just a few short decades before it was overturned within conventional medicine by new discoveries in bacteriology (though it was to live on, especially in systems of complementary and alternative medicine, among numerous publics). Nor would the old history-of-medicine regime have shown much interest in what especially intrigued Rosenberg—the sort of communication that was possible between physicians and patients when both accepted the same basic theory of how the body worked, and how health and disease came about, as unquestioned common sense. On his account, in effect, all physician–patient communication since those days represents a post-Edenic fall from grace.

When history of medicine and of illness adopts the social-history approach, a historical vantage point becomes analogous to one contribution that the study of literature makes to medicine and to bioethics. Alice Walker's short story "Strong Horse Tea" allows me to see life from the vantage point of a poor black Southern mother, perhaps with mental disabilities, whose child is dying of a treatable infection during the middle of the twentieth century.[40] Once my eyes have been opened to that vantage point, I am no longer free to go back to seeing any of the relevant issues in quite the same way I had previously—when, through ignorance, I was unable to imagine how the world would look to such a person (or that the ideas or views of such a person were worth considering). Similarly, once I have seen how the world looked, and why it looked that way, to sufferers from cholera in Paris in 1832, or to the physicians who treated them, or to the sanitary reformers who were trying to control and prevent such epidemic outbreaks, I no longer can view today's medical thinking on many subjects with the same air of unquestioning scientific privilege that I previously attributed to it.

I must now accept two possibilities alongside my allegiance to the thinking of my own day and place. First, I must acknowledge that people once thought very differently from the way I do, and yet, by all meaningful standards, they were both intelligent and rational. Second, I have to consider the possibility (actually the near-certainty) that in 100 or 150 or perhaps many fewer years, what I think today will be scoffed at as primitive by the expert thinkers of that future medicine, for reasons that I cannot even vaguely fathom.

History thus provides bioethics with an alternative vantage point, the critical distance needed at times to call previously unquestioned suppositions into dispute. The same lessons in humility that can usefully be taught to physicians are of value to bioethicists too.

## :: Religion

I believe that virtues are an important aspect of bioethics. I also believe that *forgiveness* is critical if we are to expect that health professionals become ideally virtuous. The ability to forgive others, and the ability to forgive oneself, are closely allied. Self-forgiveness is an essential ingredient in virtue. Trying to become progressively more virtuous over time—a basic demand of virtue, properly understood—means inevitably that we will frequently fall short of our goals. If we could not forgive ourselves for these lapses of virtue, it is unlikely that we would become properly motivated to continue to pursue virtue.

To the best of my recollection, I did not learn what I say here about *forgiveness* from any philosophical or specifically bioethical source. The importance of forgiveness was brought to my attention through dialogue with colleagues trained primarily in religion.[41] If so, this is just one example of why bioethics needs regular dialogue with religion and religious ethics to thrive.[42]

Any review of the history of U.S. bioethics would make it appear odd that we even have to speak today of reclaiming opportunities for bioethics and religion to speak to each other. In the early 1970s, the two towering figures in American medical ethics were the liberal author of *Situation Ethics*, Joseph Fletcher, and the conservative theologian Paul Ramsey. While often refusing to share the same stage with each other, each man would have been very comfortable describing himself as a teacher of Christian ethics. The Society for Health and Human Values, the first national organization that included those who taught bioethics in medical schools, began as a society of ministers in medical education.[43]

Later, scholars coming into bioethics from a background in religion, religious studies, or religious ethics appeared to go in one of two general directions. Some, while remaining very comfortable in departments of religion, spoke and wrote almost exclusively in a secular voice. These scholars, perhaps, viewed health professionals as their intended audience, and were aware that health professionals came from a wide variety of religious faiths (or none at all). It might well have seemed disrespectful, to these scholars, to try to address their audience in explicitly religious language, so long as the key ethical concepts they wished to discuss could appropriately be presented in secular terms.

Others thought it important to retain their explicitly religious voices, but chose to address themselves to fellow members of their faith communities. So we had Catholic bioethics textbooks and journals for Catholics, Jewish bioethics textbooks and journals for Jews, and so on. No doubt, these scholars wished that people outside of the faith community would read what they had to say, as each religious faith transmits a body of wisdom that is generally enlightening to human society, quite apart from its role as a sectarian teaching. But that is not, in practice, what happened. So the larger community of bioethics tended to tune out what these "denominational" scholars were saying.

As a result, the religious ethicists who were seen as participating most fully in the larger bioethics enterprise did not sound very religious; and those who sounded most religious appeared to be, in a sense, withdrawing from the general bioethics world to live in a cloistered corner of it. The result appeared (in this over-simplified depiction) to be a separation between religion and bioethics.[44]

One indirect way to reduce the chasm between religion and bioethics is to insist upon a closer alliance between medicine and religion than is usually supposed. David Barnard makes just such a claim in an important paper called, "The Physician as Priest, Revisited." Barnard admits that there are many compelling reasons to be suspicious of invoking for physicians anything resembling a "priestly role," and that such a role has in the past led to unfortunate abuses of power. Nevertheless, Barnard insists:

> Faith, mystery, and religion are vital elements in human suffering and medical practice. Illness is more than a biophysical event. It is also an existential crisis, with psychological, social, and spiritual dimensions in both its onset and its amelioration. Though it would be intellectually tidy and professionally convenient to draw a clean line between biophysical and "psycho-spiritual" needs in human illness, suffering persons do not present themselves that way. The physician's healing activities do incorporate ministerial functions.[45]

Barnard goes on to develop an insightful analogy between the minister and the physician. Both are mediators; both represent a power that they do not actually possess. The minister's special appeal to the parishioner is that, on one hand, she represents a higher power, the divine. In a small way, she is divinity brought down to earth to walk among humans. At the same time, she is herself a fellow, fallible human being, who can sympathize with all the parishioner's weaknesses and vulnerabilities. The physician, at least one not suffering from a God complex, analogously represents in human form the impersonal power of medical science. The physician, at the same time, is a fellow human, who can (or ought to be able to) empathically experience the patient's bodily and spiritual suffering. Barnard adds that the trust placed in the minister/physician by the parishioner/patient is a sort of gift, without which neither would have the practical power to heal suffering: "Ministry as a vocation is thus also a life of indebtedness for empowerment."[46] Physicians, he reminds us, would do well to keep in mind this basic fact of indebtedness, of reciprocity in the relationship with the patient.

Perhaps medicine can be more closely allied to religion, or ministry, without suggesting that bioethics ought to be so allied. Barnard goes on to remind us that the minister has a prophetic as well as a pastoral role. He urges physicians to adopt a stronger role of public advocacy and to accept a mantle of the prophetic role with regard to three idolatries that he finds prevalent in modern life: the idolatry of technology, the idolatry of the marketplace, and the idolatry of the nation-state (referring here to the dangers of nuclear holocaust).[47] If physicians are called upon to advocate in this way, it would certainly seem appropriate for bioethics to help them find their voice for the task.[48]

Ronald Carson is another author who has come to bioethics initially via religion. He suggests that those who see a substantial gulf between religion and bioethics might be seeing only one form of theology, systematic theology, which "aims to systematize and defend propositional statements of faith arising from communities of faith." He reminds us of an alternative that William F. May labeled "problematic theology," which "joins practitioners of other humanities disciplines in sorting through experience and trying to make livable sense of it."[49] Problematic theology applied to bioethics requires "an interpretive grasp of the manner in which morality is embedded in practices and of the ways in which communities of practice are guided by living traditions of thought and conduct."[50]

One might imagine that Carson is here simply recapitulating the debate for and against principlism in bioethics, and claiming that problematic theology is an antidote to principlism. Elsewhere, he criticizes bioethics for the way that "the bulk of the writing in the field continues to be predicated on the vision of a society populated by self-determined individuals whose mutual relations are driven by rational self-interest and governed by negotiated consent."[51] If that is Carson's brief, then one could object that he has no need to turn to theology and religion. Philosophical ethics has developed plenty of tools to oppose principlism, including casuistic, particularistic, and narrative approaches to bioethics. But Carson goes on, "We late moderns are in a moral muddle, not for epistemological reasons, but because we are spiritually adrift. It is not that we are faithless, and thus in need of moral prescriptions, but that we are having trouble understanding our moral sentiments and convictions well enough to live by them."[52] Carson admits that problematic theology is not *uniquely* suited to address our spiritual malaise. All the humanities disciplines have tools that can be brought to bear. Nonetheless, theology of the sort that he advocates has a good track record; it can hit the ground running, so to speak.

These thoughts lead Carson to return to one of the ways religion "disappeared" into bioethics—when ethical insights initially expressed in theological terms were translated into secular language. What was lost in the translation? Carson gives as an example the way that some might have thought that the essential content of Paul Ramsey's *The Patient as Person* emerged unscathed, and indeed better fleshed out, in the principle of respect for autonomy. Yet something was lost with "the collapsing of Ramsey's robust covenantal notion of 'awesome respect' for persons" into the much less morally dense language of self-determination.[53]

Let me extend this suggestion more generally. Based on my limited understanding of the religious, what bioethics leaves out, when it tries to go about its business without cross-talk with religion, is a sense of *awe* and of *mystery*—the basic human response to what we perceive to be much larger than ourselves. Bioethics, like medicine, tends to want to turn all mysteries into puzzles, so that solutions will be forthcoming. Barnard quotes Paul Pruyser's observation about responding to human suffering: "the religious essence does not lie in the answer but in taking the question seriously and with compassion."[54]

Closely tied to awe and mystery, religion often focuses on how we go about attaching *meaning* to the world and to events that happen to us and around us. When bioethics is doing ethical or policy analysis, we tend to imagine that the meaning of the variables is already given. *If* things mean what they mean, *then* it follows that we ought to take certain actions. Religion may be more open than secular bioethics to the awareness that we *create* meaning by our choices and actions. James Childress may be pointing to this aspect of religion when he suggests that religion adds to ethical and policy analysis a dimension of *imagination:* "[P]ublic reasoning includes imagination, not only rational deductions from shared secular premises. Religious stories and theological concepts may enable us to imagine and re-imagine in ways that are fruitful for public policy."[55]

## ⁑ The Social Sciences

It has become routine for scholars in the medical humanities to distinguish between two kinds of social science, one excluded from, and the other incorporated into, their field. Social scientists who merely catalogue the behavior of individuals or groups are generally seen as not doing medical humanities. The social scientists included in the field are those who inquire more deeply about the meanings, values, and attitudes that underlie the behaviors.[56] In general, the methods used by these humanities-inclined social scientists are participant-observer and ethnographic studies, those that yield "thick descriptions" of human activities.[57]

A great deal could be said about what the social sciences have to offer bioethics, and what sorts of work in the social sciences will best suit these needs. By way of demonstrating what I take to be the special strengths of the social sciences in shedding new light on bioethics, I will use only one example, a study by Susan Kelly and her colleagues of the process of ethics consultation in several U.S. West Coast urban hospitals.[58]

A member of the research team, a medical student, participated in nine ethics consultations, which were all the consultations that occurred in those hospitals during the three-month study period. The consultations occurred in three different hospitals, each of which had a different structure for its ethics committee and consultation team. All available participants in the consultation were also interviewed, usually about a month after the consultation occurred.

Kelly and colleagues summarized their major findings:

> [W]e found that asymmetries in power, status, and culture were sustained in the ethics consultations observed. Ironically, the practice of ethics consultation is in part intended to help overcome this disequilibrium....

To the extent that ethics consultation provides what Walker called "those moral-reflective spaces in institutional life where a sound and shared process of deliberation and negotiation can go on," we found that these are structured moral spaces, structured in ways that reflect the hierarchical nature and power relationships of the institution and broader professional and social communities in which they are situated.[59]

The research team discovered that ethical categories and principles often seemed to have very little to do with when an ethics consultation was requested or what was the outcome. Rather, consultations appeared to function as ways to deal with conflicts that arose within the hospital when a "normal" routine was disrupted by the behavior of one or more parties. Requests for consultations by more powerful parties—notably physicians—were treated with more urgency and priority than requests from others. Members of one family, interviewed after the consultation, remained very angry at the process, describing it as "a big sham" in which they had been "railroaded," and as an opportunity for physicians to "prey upon the family's emotions" until they "broke down."[60]

This particular bit of social science research is of great interest because bioethics is, as we have seen, a working practice and not solely a collection of ideas and texts.[61] Margaret Urban Walker, in the passage cited within the research report, refers to bioethics as "moral-reflective"; and Ronald Carson characterizes medical ethics as "reflective practice."[62] As a result, bioethics may be tempted to give itself airs—the physicians and nurses and patients and families, poor benighted souls, go about their business in the hospital, driven this way and that by scientific pro-tocols, work routines, emotions, and cultural traditions. Meanwhile, we bioethicists are the reflective ones of the bunch, able to stand back and use our ethical skills and insights to probe to the root of what is really going on and what is at stake.

If we are tempted to regard ourselves in this way, then it would seem that the social scientists have done us one better and out-reflected us.[63] I very much doubt that the hospital ethics consultants in the Kelly study, asked to describe what they had done, would have characterized it in the way that the ethnographers did. Without passing judgment for the moment on which description—the ethnographers' or the consultant's—would have been "correct" (if either was), the point remains that the discussion of what actually goes on in ethics consultation is enriched immeasurably when the ethnographic description is laid on the table for consideration. The possibility that the work of ethics consultation is not merely *different from* the way it is usually described within the field of bioethics, but that it actually *undermines* important ethical values through the way that it may be practiced in some contexts, would very likely never emerge for discussion otherwise.

Studying bioethicists is only one of many functions that social scientists may perform; a larger portion of their research is devoted to studying how people respond to illness and how health-care institutions function from both the providers' and the patients' points of view. Those research findings can all be of considerable value for bioethics and medical humanities.[64] I selected the Kelly et al. study as an example precisely because it goes for the bioethical jugular. Given the important issues that the study raises, I find it quite unfortunate that so few studies of its type were performed during the decade following its publication.

It might seem that I have loaded the dice by selecting a social-science study that directly addresses a core activity in bioethics, in order to prove the relevance of the former discipline to the latter. Besides this sort of focused inquiry into bioethics-as-practice, however, the methodology of the social sciences provides a useful form of cross-talk for bioethics more generally. For the social scientist, as a rule, ethical reasoning and conduct represents merely one more example of complex human behavior. The same participant-observer methods can be employed to study a society's ethics as might be used to study how they exchange goods in the marketplace, how parents rear children, or how parishioners engage in religious rituals. Ethics, on this account, has no special status; and far less is it viewed as having any sort of conceptual purity. These fundamental differences in how ethics is seen by the different disciplines can make cross-talk extremely frustrating for both, as at first no real communication seems possible.[65] If both sides work at it, however, these initial frustrations can be overcome. Bioethicists can then discover the stimulation of being forced to rethink some of their assumptions.[66]

Raymond De Vries, who has written extensively on the interface between bioethics and sociology, sometimes seems to imagine that sociology can be most useful to bioethics when it is most domesticated— when it explores important issues in bioethics and discovers facts about human society that bioethicists can then contemplate and reason with. Sociology, he suggests, is less useful to bioethics when it attacks some of the most basic premises on which bioethics is based as being empirically uninformed or implausible. He urges us not to judge sociology solely on the basis of its usefulness to bioethics, since sociologists can in fact be doing their best work when they question the basic assumptions of our field.[67] I agree that such foundational excavations can be good sociology. But, I would add, they can also be good bioethics. A bioethics that refuses to engage in such excavations, drawing upon whatever other disciplines have the best tools for digging, is to that extent an impoverished bioethics. That is part of the reason why bioethics must remain resolutely interdisciplinary.

## ⚌ Conclusion: How Narrow and Conservative is Bioethics?

Almost every ethics consultant has had the experience of being called to a patient's bedside, rendering an ethical recommendation, and then hearing the attending physicians bellow like gored oxen: "What do you mean, we cannot just go ahead and do what we have always done in the past? What do you mean, we have to ask the patient what she wants? What do you mean, the hospital has policies that we must follow?" After a few such experiences, the bioethicist can easily come to the conclusion that she's a radical agent of change within the hospital, more likely to get into trouble by being seen by powerful medical interests as a loose cannon, than to be accused of excessive timidity.

For this bioethicist to be confronted with the charge that she's fundamentally a conservative protector of the medical status quo must, at first, be bewildering. Yet that is the picture painted by Tina Stevens, whose remit is the relationship between bioethics and history, but who calls for support for the work of social scientists Raymond De Vries and Peter Conrad. They claim that bioethics needs sociology because otherwise we are far too narrow in our perspective. We don't see the relationship between the ethical problems that we identify and the larger structure of medical care systems. Such a narrow view condemns us to ignoring structural deficiencies in health care by reinterpreting them as "ethical dilemmas." We end up inevitably serving the interests of the organization and its powerful defenders.[68]

To the bioethics consultant described above, it appears that her field has set itself apart from medicine, fully prepared to be highly critical of medical activities and ways of thinking. To Kathryn Montgomery, approaching medicine and bioethics via literature, it seems that bioethics has been bitten by the medicine bug and become infected. Medicine at the start of the twenty-first century is a uniquely positivist, reductionist enterprise. In most of the world of modern science, something of the intellectual breeze of the late twentieth century has sifted through the cracks. Scientists in many fields have a renewed appreciation for the fallacies inherent in the subjectivity/objectivity distinction, and accept that their work is awash in subjectivity in a way that their teachers' generation hardly realized. Medicine has been nearly alone among the so-called scientific fields in resisting this awareness. Held in thrall by the vital importance of its work, that of preserving human life, medicine is nearly alone in continuing to insist that it can be wholly objective.

Montgomery thinks that bioethics has become afflicted with medicine's objectivity disease, leading it to systematically ignore and devalue its own necessary reliance on subjectivity:

> Demands for answers in the real world of clinical problems and public policy—like the effect on physicians of similar demands in the care of patients—has kept most medical ethicists focused on topical questions. The commodification of health care and the undiminished acceleration of medical technology—the human genome project, transgenic xenotransplantation, cloning—have meant that philosophers in medicine, though moderately radical when they depart from mainstream philosophy to take up real-world questions, still hold as essential and unquestioned the analytic tools they learned as graduate students....[Q]uestions of subjectivity and the ethics of representation have been almost entirely neglected in medical ethics. In this it resembles medicine, but without medicine's modernist, practical excuse.[69]

Montgomery goes on to catalogue the specific weaknesses of philosophically grounded bioethics: "a reluctance to see knowledge as inevitably situated and contextual, a rush to judgment on questions of policy and practice that neglects the opportunity to educate participants, a lack of interest in the relation of its theory to its practice, and a widely held assumption that emotion is irrational. All stem from the monocular privileging of logico-mathematical rationality.... The result is the failure of an intellectual (and too often a practical) interdisciplinarity."[70] If bioethics were truly to address its weaknesses, we would all be taking more seriously questions posed by Hilde Lindemann Nelson—How can an ethicist honor the personal without being arbitrary? and John Arras—How can we "acknowledge our individuality and situatedness without abandoning the possibility of social criticism"?[71]

It is critically important to bioethics' practical agenda whether or not Montgomery has described the problem accurately. As she has already mentioned, a failure of interdisciplinarity is a practical as well as an intellectual problem. If bioethics is heavily invested in defending medicine's current power structure—and yet does not realize that it is so invested—then it seems vain to hope that bioethics can ever assume an activist posture, and help those now without power to raise their own voices and be heard.

There is another highly practical question related to these concerns about interdisciplinarity. Where, as the vulgar phrase has it, should bioethicists hang out? If "cross-talk" among the disciplines is truly necessary for the enterprise, then bioethicists, it would seem, should rub shoulders with these colleagues on a more or less regular basis. How does one make this happen? How should a bioethics program be structured to encourage this—even at the mundane level of designing the office space?

Montgomery offers her own home discipline of literary studies as the reasonable antidote to all the ills she has identified. As we have seen in this chapter, all of the disciplines we have surveyed offer something of value in amending bioethics' narrowness of vision and tendencies toward conservatism. Bioethics, construed as (philosophical) ethics plus medicine and the biological sciences, is by its nature interdisciplinary—but not enough so.[72] It needs the other humanities and related social-science disciplines to flourish.

NOTES TO CHAPTER 2

1. Jennings B. Traumatic brain injury and the goals of care. The ordeal of reminding. *Hastings Cent Rep* 36(2):29–37, 2006; Hoffmaster B. What does vulnerability mean? *Hastings Cent Rep* 36(2):38–45, 2006.
2. One might argue that in my selection of authors, I have slanted the "data" in my preferred interdisciplinary direction. Barry Hoffmaster holds a Ph.D. in philosophy and teaches in a university philosophy department; so it may be "news" that he would offer a narrative rather than an analytical account. Bruce Jennings, by contrast, holds a masters degree in political science. He is quite capable of work that analytical philosophers would consider as part of their field—see, for instance, my discussion in Chapter 5 of his arguments on democratic consensus. Still, he could be viewed as by nature a more interdisciplinary sort of person, having migrated as it were from political science into bioethics.
3. In a commentary on Jennings, Marilyn Martone argues that even he offers an overly idealistic picture of what is possible; Martone M. Traumatic brain injury and the goals of care. *Hastings Cent Rep* 36(2):3, 2006.
4. Macklin R. The new conservatives in bioethics: who are they and what do they seek? *Hastings Cent Rep* 36(1):34–43, 2006; Cohen E. Conservative bioethics and the search for wisdom. *Hastings Cent Rep* 36(1):44–56, 2006.
5. President's Council on Bioethics. *Taking care: ethical caregiving in our aging society.* Washington, DC: President's Council on Bioethics, 2005.
6. Jeffrey Kahn and Anna Mastroianni begin their editorial introduction to a special journal issue on "the future of bioethics" by stating that,

"Bioethics is a necessarily interdisciplinary and multidisciplinary field"; Kahn J, Mastroianni A. Introduction: looking forward in bioethics. *J Law Med Ethics* 32:196–97, 2004.

7. Earlier, Jennings and Hoffmaster had been singled out as bioethicists who had a special predilection toward ethnographic approaches to their field; De Vries R, Conrad P. Why bioethics needs sociology. In: De Vries R, Subedi J, eds. *Bioethics and society: constructing the ethical enterprise*. Upper Saddle River, NJ: Prentice-Hall, 1998, pp. 233–57, esp. pp. 248–50.

8. Judith Andre argues that all practical ethics, let alone bioethics, is interdisciplinary by its very nature. Ultimately, ethics is about what has value; and no single discipline has a corner on the market of illuminating for us what has value and why. She offers this account as an antidote especially to anyone who would argue that ethics is best understood solely as a subfield within philosophy. Andre J. *Bioethics as practice*. Chapel Hill, NC: University of North Carolina Press, 2002, pp. 68–9.

9. Martensen R. Thought styles among the medical humanities: past, present, and near-term future. In: Carson RA, Burns CR, Cole TR, eds. *Practicing the medical humanities: engaging physicians and patients*. Hagerstown, MD: University Publishing Group, 2003, pp. 99–122. Those who find "cross-talk" insufficiently titillating may be moved to follow Haavi Morreim's suggestion: Morreim EH. At the intersection of medicine, law, economics, and ethics: bioethics and the art of intellectual cross-dressing. In: Carson RA, Burns CR, eds. *Philosophy of medicine and bioethics*. Boston: Kluwer Academic Publishers, 1997, pp. 299–325. (I am grateful to William Winslade for reminding me of this paper; see also Winslade WJ. Intellectual cross-dressing: an eccentricity or a practical necessity? Commentary on Morreim. In: Carson RA, Burns CR, eds. *Philosophy of medicine and bioethics*, pp. 327–34.) It is important to note that the present chapter is not intended to be a discussion of the nature or value of the medical humanities. Each of the disciplines I survey has a great deal to offer to an understanding of medicine, quite apart from what it can accomplish in conjunction with bioethics.

10. For one more comprehensive listing of disciplines contributing to bioethics, see: Miller FG, Fletcher JC, Humber JM, eds. *The nature and prospect of bioethics: interdisciplinary perspectives*. Totowa, NJ: Humana Press, 2003. I have elected not to include philosophy in this chapter because (perhaps due to my own training in that discipline) I simply assume that the relationship between bioethics and philosophical ethics is both obvious and unassailable. I cannot agree with Pellegrino that the tie between philosophical ethics and bioethics is under threat, though whether philosophy provides a "foundation" for bioethics is quite another matter: Pellegrino ED. Bioethics as an interdisciplinary enterprise: where does ethics fit in the mosaic of disciplines? In: Carson RA, Burns CR, eds. *Philosophy of medicine and bioethics*, pp. 1–23.

11. An excellent brief overview of narrative ethics is given by Jones AH. Narrative based medicine: narrative in medical ethics. *BMJ* 318:253–56, 1999. My own previous work has in some ways illustrated the progress of

this concept. In the first edition of *Stories of Sickness*, I addressed primarily the importance of narrative for understanding sickness and medicine, and touched very lightly on the notion of narrative ethics: *Stories of sickness*. New Haven, CT: Yale University Press, 1987. A few years later I elaborated one of the suggestive notions in the book, that of a "relational ethics" of medicine: "My story is broken, can you help me fix it?" Medical ethics and the joint construction of narrative. *Lit Med* 13:79–92, 1994. Finally, I attempted a more systematic treatment of narrative ethics: *Stories of sickness*, 2nd ed. New York: Oxford University Press, 2003.

12. Jones AH. Narrative based medicine: narrative in medical ethics. *BMJ* 318:253–56, 1999. The principal proponent of "narrative approaches to bioethics," according to Jones's distinction, is Rita Charon. See, for instance, Charon R. Narrative contributions to medical ethics: recognition, formulation, interpretation, and validation in the practice of the ethicist. In: DuBose ER, Hamel RP, O'Connell LJ, eds. *A matter of principles? Ferment in U.S. bioethics*. Valley Forge, PA: Trinity Press International, 1994, pp. 260–83; and Charon R. *Narrative medicine: honoring the stories of illness*. New York: Oxford University Press, 2006.

13. Charon R. *Narrative medicine: honoring the stories of illness*, p. 53.

14. This critical question is posed by Arthur Frank; Frank A. *The wounded storyteller: body, illness, and ethics*. Chicago: University of Chicago Press, 1995, pp.158–63.

15. Brody H. *Stories of sickness*, 2nd ed., pp.172–272.

16. Johnson M. *Moral imagination: implications of cognitive science for ethics*. Chicago: University of Chicago Press, 1993.

17. Walker MU. *Moral understandings: a feminist study in ethics*. New York: Routledge, 1998.

18. Brody H. *Stories of sickness*, 2nd ed., pp. 201–3.

19. "'Literature,' writes Louise Rosenblatt, 'provides a *living through*, not simply *knowledge about*,' suggesting that the reader does not remain untouched through the act of reading but rather becomes open to fundamental transformation by virtue of having read." Charon R. *Narrative medicine: honoring the stories of illness*, p. 57, citing in turn Rosenblatt LM. *Literature as exploration*. New York: Modern Language Association, 1995, p. 38.

20. Nelson HL. *Damaged identities, narrative repair*. Ithaca, NY: Cornell University Press, 2001; Nelson HL. Feminist bioethics: where we've been, where we're going. *Metaphilosophy* 31:492–508, 2000.

21. Montgomery K. Medical ethics: literature, literary studies, and the question of interdisciplinarity. In: Miller FG, Fletcher JC, Humber JM, eds. *The nature and prospect of bioethics: interdisciplinary perspectives*. Totowa, NJ: Humana Press, 2003, pp. 141–78, quote on p. 169.

22. Arras J. Nice story, but so what? narrative and justification in ethics. In: Nelson HL, ed. *Stories and their limits: narrative approaches to bioethics*. New York: Routledge, 1997, pp. 65–88, quote on p. 83.

23. Chambers T. *The fiction of bioethics: cases as literary texts*. New York: Routledge, 1999.

24. Montgomery K. Medical ethics: literature, literary studies, and the question of interdisciplinarity. In: Miller FG, Fletcher JC, Humber JM, eds. *The nature and prospect of bioethics: interdisciplinary perspectives*, pp. 141–78. She cites in turn Banks JT. Literature as a clinical capacity: commentary on "the Quasimodo Complex." *J Clin Ethics* 1:227–31, 1990; and Hawkins AH. Literature, medical ethics, and epiphanic knowledge. *J Clin Ethics* 5:283–90, 1994.

25. Veatch RM. *Disrupted dialogue: medical ethics and the collapse of physician–humanist communication* (1770–1980). New York: Oxford University Press, 2005.

26. However, for charges that Veatch fell short in the area of historical accuracy, see Latham SR. Review of Robert M. Veatch, Disrupted dialogue: medical ethics and the collapse of physician–humanist dialogue, 1770–1980. *Am J Bioethics* 7:95–96, 2007.

27. Ryan M. *Manual of medical jurisprudence*, 2nd ed. London: Sherwood, Gilbert and Piper, 1836.

28. Baker RB, McCullough LB. Introduction. In: Baker RB, McCullough LB, eds. *Cambridge world history of medical ethics*. New York: Cambridge University Press, in press.

29. See, for example, Zuger A, Miles SH. Physicians, AIDS, and occupational risk: historical traditions and ethical obligations. *JAMA* 258:1924–28, 1987.

30. See, for example, Veatch RM *Case studies in medical ethics*. Cambridge, MA: Harvard University Press, 1977; Veatch RM. Professional ethics: new principles for physicians. *Hastings Cent Rep* 10(3):16–19, 1980; Veatch RM. *Death, dying and the biological revolution: our last quest for responsibility*. New Haven, CT: Yale University Press, 1989.

31. A related argument for ignoring such works as those of Gregory and Percival was that these earlier authors were not doing medical *ethics* in any meaningful sense; their works were rather about medical *etiquette;* Leake CD. Preface. In: *Percival's medical ethics*. Baltimore: Williams and Wilkins, 1927. It now seems clear that this argument was based on an anachronistic reading of those texts; see, for example, Haakonssen L. *Medicine and morals in the Enlightenment: John Gregory, Thomas Percival, and Benjamin Rush*. Atlanta: Rodopi, 1997.

32. Bioethicists might reject history for yet another reason, pointed out by Tina Stevens—that ultimately, historians have no stake whatever in whether bioethics succeeds or fails: "For chroniclers, accounting for how and why bioethics declined would be as irresistible a project as explaining its genesis and growth." Stevens MLT. History and bioethics. In: Miller FG, Fletcher JC, Humber JM, eds. *The nature and prospect of bioethics: interdisciplinary perspectives*, pp. 179–96, quote on pp. 179–80.

33. Historians are probably less well represented at meetings of the American Society for Bioethics and Humanities than any comparable humanities discipline; and the meetings of the ASBH affinity group on "History of Medical Ethics" are relatively sparsely attended.

34. Rothman D. *Strangers at the bedside: a history of how law and bioethics transformed medical decision making*. New York: Basic Books, 1991.

Tina Stevens makes the helpful suggestion that some of bioethics' modern roots may be found in the responsible-use-of-science movement that grew up in the 1950s in reaction to nuclear weapons, and that was later extended to the new genetics; Stevens MLT. *Bioethics in America: origins and cultural politics.* Baltimore: Johns Hopkins University Press, 2000. Stevens's analysis is flawed by her penchant for trying to identify a *single* historical explanation for most phenomena in bioethics and rejecting accounts that propose alternative explanations. For a critical review of Stevens's book, see Jonsen AR Beating up bioethics [review essay]. *Hastings Cent Rep* 31(5):40–45, 2001.

35. McCullough LB, ed. *John Gregory and the invention of professional medical ethics and the profession of medicine.* Boston: Kluwer Academic Publishers, 1998.

36. Haakonssen L. *Medicine and morals in the Enlightenment: John Gregory, Thomas Percival, and Benjamin Rush.* Atlanta: Rodopi, 1997.

37. Percival T. *Medical ethics; or, a code of institutes and precepts adapted to the professional conduct of physicians and surgeons...* Manchester, England: Russell, 1803; modern reprint by the Classics of Medicine Library, Birmingham, AL, 1985, pp. 156–68.

38. Martensen R. Thought styles among the medical humanities: past, present, and near-term future. In: Carson RA, Burns CR, Cole TR, eds. *Practicing the medical humanities: engaging physicians and patients.* Hagerstown, MD: University Publishing Group, 2003, pp. 99–122.

39. Rosenberg CE. The therapeutic revolution: medicine, meaning, and social change in nineteenth century America. In: Vogel MJ, Rosenberg CE, eds. *The therapeutic revolution: essays in the social history of American medicine.* Philadelphia: University of Pennsylvania Press, 1979, pp. 3–25.

40. Walker A. Strong horse tea. In: Secundy MG, Nixon LL, eds. *Trials, tribulations, and celebrations: African-American perspectives on health, illness, aging and loss.* Yarmouth, ME: Intercultural Press, 1992, pp. 76–82.

41. I am especially indebted to my former colleagues at Michigan State University who directed the course in spirituality and health—first, Fr. John P. "Jake" Foglio; and subsequently, the Rev. Clayton Thomason. Fr. Foglio's standard example on self-forgiveness went, "If I get up in church and give a sermon on any subject, I can be sure that I will violate at least one thing that I said in that sermon within the next 24 hours." To go on functioning as a priest, he needed to be able to forgive himself for those predictable lapses. He insisted that self-forgiveness ought not lead to complacency, and that rather, it could coexist with determined efforts to improve one's future performance.

42. Daniel Callahan commented, "Though I am not myself religious, I consider the decline of religious contributions [to bioethics] a misfortune, leading to a paucity of concepts, a thin imagination, and the ignorance of traditions, practices, and forms of moral analysis of great value"; Callahan D. The social sciences and the task of bioethics. *Daedalus* 128:275–94, 1999, quote on p. 280.

43. The Society for Health and Human Values was formed in 1968. In 1998 it merged with the Society for Bioethics Consultation and the American Association of Bioethics to form the American Society for Bioethics and Humanities. James Childress challenges this "myth" of bioethics having its recent origin in religion, and then becoming gradually more secularized, but I am unable to follow his reasoning completely; Childress JF. Religion, theology and bioethics. In: Miller FG, Fletcher JC, Humber JM, eds. *The nature and prospect of bioethics: interdisciplinary perspectives*, pp. 43–67.

44. It is important to note that this separation may have been a uniquely American phenomenon. Michael Selgelid, for instance, of Sydney, Australia, in a paper prepared for the VI World Congress of Bioethics in Brasilia, 2002, spoke deprecatingly of the "hijacking" of the bioethics debate by religion. In his view, religion has played a largely conservative and unhelpful role in bioethics, in the form of objections to abortion, euthanasia, stem-cell research, and so on; Selgelid MJ. Ethics and infectious disease. *Bioethics* 19:272–89, 2005. On a visit to Argentina in 1995, several South American bioethicists told me confidentially that their work was rendered much more difficult by the near-absolute requirement that they say nothing that would offend the powerful Catholic church authorities. British bioethicists have told me that the relatively slow development of the field in the United Kingdom, compared to the United States, was due to the need for British bioethics to emerge from under the shadow of the Anglican Church; until it had clearly separated itself in the minds of physicians, any bioethical discourse was viewed as a Sunday sermon, to be ignored by pragmatic professionals.

45. Barnard D. The physician as priest, revisited. *J Religion Health* 24:272–86, 1985, quote on p. 278.

46. Barnard D. The physician as priest, revisited, quote on p. 280.

47. Barnard D. The physician as priest, revisited, quote on p. 284.

48. According to James Childress's review of the role of religion in bioethics, James Gustafson had initially proposed that bioethics had four distinct voices—narrative, ethical analysis, policy, and prophetic; Childress JF. Religion, theology and bioethics. In: Miller FG, Fletcher JC, Humber JM, eds. *The nature and prospect of bioethics: interdisciplinary perspectives*, pp. 43–67. The narrative voice seems to overlap the domain of literature and medicine, though we should be open to the realization that there are peculiarly religious aspects and forms of narrative. Of these four, the prophetic voice would seem most suggestive of a link with religion, though religious scholars could still add unique contributions to bioethics as ethical analysis.

49. Carson RA. Focusing on the human scene. Thoughts on problematic theology. In: Davis DS, Zoloth L, eds. *Notes from a narrow ridge: religion and bioethics*. Hagerstown, MD: University Publishing Group, 1999, pp. 49–63, quotes on p. 50.

50. Carson RA. Focusing on the human scene. Thoughts on problematic theology, quote on p. 52.

51. Carson RA. Medical ethics as reflective practice. In: Carson RA, Burns CR, eds. *Philosophy of medicine and bioethics*. Boston: Kluwer Academic Publishers, 1997:181–91, quote on p. 182.

52. Carson RA. Focusing on the human scene. Thoughts on problematic theology, quote on p. 53.

53. Carson RA. Focusing on the human scene. Thoughts on problematic theology, quote on p. 55.

54. Barnard D. The physician as priest, revisited. *J Religion Health* 24:272–86, 1985, quote on p. 282. The original source is Pruyser PW. *A dynamic psychology of religion*. New York: Harper and Row, 1968, p. 215.

55. Childress JF. Religion, theology and bioethics. In: Miller FG, Fletcher JC, Humber JM, eds. *The nature and prospect of bioethics: interdisciplinary perspectives,* pp. 43–67, quote on p. 60.

56. A thoughtful discussion of the relationship between anthropology and bioethics is Marshall PA. Anthropology and bioethics. *Med Anthropol Q* 6:49–73, 1992. Another social scientist whose work has been widely accepted and endorsed by bioethicists is Charles Bosk; Bosk CL. *Forgive and remember: managing medical failure*. Chicago: University of Chicago Press, 1979; Bosk CL. *All God's mistakes: genetic counseling in a pediatric hospital*. Chicago: University of Chicago Press, 1992.

57. Geertz C. *The interpretation of cultures*. New York: Basic Books, 1973; Davis DS. Rich cases: the ethics of thick description. *Hastings Cent Rep* 21(4):12–17, 1991.

58. Kelly SE, Marshall PA, Sanders LM, et al. Understanding the process of ethics consultation: results of an ethnographic multi-site study. *J Clin Ethics* 8:136–49, 1997.

59. Kelly SE, Marshall PA, Sanders LM, et al. Understanding the process of ethics consultation: results of an ethnographic multi-site study, quote on p. 145. The reference within the quotation is to Walker MU. Keeping moral space open: new images of ethics consulting. *Hastings Cent Rep* 23(2):33–40, 1993, quote on p. 38.

60. Kelly SE, Marshall PA, Sanders LM, et al. Understanding the process of ethics consultation: results of an ethnographic multi-site study, quote on p. 143.

61. Andre J. *Bioethics as practice*. Chapel Hill, NC: University of North Carolina Press, 2002:

62. Walker MU. Keeping moral space open: new images of ethics consulting. *Hastings Cent Rep* 23(2):33–40, 1993; Carson RA. Medical ethics as reflective practice. In: Carson RA, Burns CR, eds. *Philosophy of medicine and bioethics,* pp. 181–91.

63. Having cited both Margaret Urban Walker and Ronald Carson on the "reflective" nature of bioethics, I must immediately add that neither would accept that bioethics has some corner on the "reflection" market and that the bioethicist is in that sense superior to other actors in the hospital "case."

64. See, for example, Turner L. Bioethics in a multicultural world: medicine and morality in pluralistic settings. *Health Care Analysis* 11:99–117, 2003.

65. Raymond De Vries offers both a historical overview of the relationship between sociology and bioethics, as well as a warning against judging sociology too much on the basis of its "usefulness" to bioethics; De Vries R. How can we help? From "sociology in" to "sociology of" bioethics. *J Law Med Ethics* 32:279–92, 2004.

66. That bioethics has begun to realize the importance of placing empirical methodology side by side with conceptual analysis is illustrated by the increasing appearance within the literature of empirical studies of behavior and attitudes. Of late, people with bioethics training who also possess skills in empirical research methodology are highly sought after as junior faculty in bioethics programs, though the reason may have more to do with their ability to secure grant funding than with an abiding appreciation for the value of their research. Sadly, the vast bulk of this literature employs survey-questionnaire methods, rather than the participant-observer methods that might better discern the interpretations and meanings the actors attribute to their behavior.

67. De Vries R. How can we help? From "sociology in" to "sociology of" bioethics. J Law Med Ethics 32:279–92, 2004. Anthropologists Patricia Marshall and Barbara Koenig add here that while bioethics has great need of input from the social sciences, bioethics must not allow itself to be undermined by the empirical and necessarily non-normative approach of the social sciences; Marshall P, Koenig B. Accounting for culture in a globalized bioethics. *J Law Med Ethics* 32:252–66, 2004. They quote with approval Daniel Callahan, that social science methods are useful "only if they are combined with a way of pursuing ethical analysis that knows how to make good use of social-science knowledge....Ethics must, in the end, be ethics, not social science"; Callahan D. The social sciences and the task of bioethics. *Daedalus* 128(4):275–94, 1999, quote on p. 283.

68. Stevens MLT. History and bioethics. In: Miller FG, Fletcher JC, Humber JM, eds. *The nature and prospect of bioethics: interdisciplinary perspectives*, pp. 179–96. Stevens in turn cites De Vries R, Conrad P. Why bioethics needs sociology. In: De Vries R, Subedi J, eds. *Bioethics and society: constructing the ethical enterprise.* Upper Saddle River, NJ: Prentice-Hall, 1998, pp. 233–57.

69. Montgomery K. Medical ethics: literature, literary studies, and the question of interdisciplinarity. In: Miller FG, Fletcher JC, Humber JM, eds. *The nature and prospect of bioethics: interdisciplinary perspectives*, pp. 141–78, quote on pp. 158–59, 161.

70. Montgomery K. Medical ethics: literature, literary studies, and the question of interdisciplinarity. Miller FG, Fletcher JC, Humber JM, eds. *The nature and prospect of bioethics: interdisciplinary perspectives*, pp. 141–78, quote on p. 165.

71. Montgomery K. Medical ethics: literature, literary studies, and the question of interdisciplinarity. In: Miller FG, Fletcher JC, Humber JM, eds. *The nature and prospect of bioethics: interdisciplinary perspectives*, pp. 141–78. Montgomery cites in turn Nelson HL. Introduction: how to do things with stories. In: Nelson HL, ed. *Stories and their limits: narrative approaches*

*to bioethics.* New York: Routledge, 1997: vii-xx. Arras J. Nice story, but so what? narrative and justification in ethics. In: Nelson HL, ed. *Stories and their limits: narrative approaches to bioethics.* pp. 65–88, quote on p. 84.

72. The notion that "bioethics" is the same thing as "the ethics of medicine and the biological sciences" is actually only one way to view the field, and, I will argue in Chapter 10, an unfortunately limited way. See the portion of Chapter 10 that deals with the "Potter Tradition" in bioethics.

# 3 ⠂⠂
# Patient-Centered Care

Sylvia Stultz, who died of a rare form of disseminated sarcoma in June, 2006, was a clinical psychologist who taught social skills to autistic children. As she went in and out of hospitals and clinics while seeking treatment for her cancer, she discovered a new calling. She found herself trying to teach social skills to health-care workers instead.

As recounted by her friend Susan Okie, a journalist and contributing editor to the *New England Journal of Medicine,* Ms. Stultz on one occasion visited the surgical oncology clinic at the Clinical Center of the National Institutes of Health in Bethesda, Maryland. She reported to the clinic, as she had been instructed, at 10:15 A.M. When, after waiting several hours, she began to ask for estimates of when she might be seen, the staff seemed puzzled that she would ask such a question. She finally met the specialist she was supposed to see at 3:30 P.M.

At the conclusion of her visit, which was quite satisfactory from a technical point of view, Ms. Stultz asked the physician why patients were kept waiting that long. Susan Okie, who was present, described the physician as "contrite," but he insisted that he had no control over scheduling matters. So Ms. Stultz wrote a letter to the director of the Clinical Center, John I. Gallin. The response was immediate and significant. Gallin called in department heads, and soon the NIH was embarked on a campaign to reduce waiting times. Gallin later told Okie, "It wasn't really obvious to me how much of a problem it was until [Ms. Stultz] sort of hit me between the eyes with a two-by-four."

A surgical implantation of radioactive needles to treat another tumor brought Ms. Stultz to the Brigham and Women's Hospital in Boston. She was told she would be immobile and in a state of near-isolation, as both nurses and visitors would have to limit time in her room due to the radioactivity risks. She counted on being distracted by her iPod, but the device was either lost or stolen between the admissions desk and her room. The night after the surgery, she awoke in intense pain. After she was already under anesthesia, the anesthesiologist had abruptly changed the planned-for program of pain control. Ms. Stultz sobbed for two hours until a nurse responded to her call, and was told that the nurse had been busy with an "emergency." Finally, Ms. Stultz was discharged with painful bedsores from lying still for three days, and was given no instructions on how to care for them at home.

When she complained of this treatment, Brigham and Women's Hospital was much less responsive than the NIH Clinical Center had been. Ms. Stultz was referred to an ombudsman, who investigated and sent her a written report after several months. Her radiation oncologist was very guarded in speaking with her, but finally unbent enough to admit that there was a "culture" in the hospital, whose origins she did not understand.[1]

If we asked a representative panel of bioethicists to rank their field's top accomplishments in the United States in the last three decades, it is hard to imagine that they would *not* place near the top of their list the replacement of the traditional deference to physician paternalism with the ascendency of the principle of respect for patient autonomy.

Try telling that to Sylvia Stultz, or to Susan Okie.

The NIH Clinical Center and Brigham and Women's Hospital (the latter a teaching affiliate of Harvard Medical School) are considered to be among the premier health facilities in the world. Both, besides boasting first-class medical staffs, have active ethics committees and teaching programs. If it were suggested to the head of the ethics program at either facility that the institution did not have a commitment to "respect for patient autonomy," I'd expect that person to object strenuously, and point to reams of official hospital policies on informed consent and similar patients'-rights issues. If asked whether the ethics program had ever considered the matter of how long patients had to wait in clinics, or if they were discharged frustrated and frightened and without adequate instructions, I'd expect the answer to be either frank puzzlement, or the objection that those are not proper "ethics issues" for the program or the committee to consider. Presumably such matters as caused distress for Ms. Stultz are somebody else's business, not that of the ethics program, if they are anyone's business at all. I do not recall having seen such matters receiving space in any standard textbook of bioethics.

Following Hilde Lindemann's query of whether we should see bio-ethics as gendered masculine or feminine, we might suspect that this is an example of bioethics wishing to appear macho.[2] Deciding on whether people live or die, whether or not to disconnect the ventilator in the ICU, appears to be a commendably masculine activity that bioethics can be proud of in medicine's masculine world. By contrast, worrying about how long it takes to be seen for one's appointment, or whether one's pain, anxieties, and needs for information were addressed, seems distressingly like "housekeeping" or "women's work." Bioethics runs a serious risk of losing status within medicine if it tries to take on those latter functions.

Lately, increasing attention is being paid within primary-care medicine to "patient-centered care" and to the related concept of a "medical home." To my knowledge, bioethicists have paid scant attention to these developments, to the extent that they are aware of them at all. It would seem, however, that a movement called "patient-centered care" should be of considerable bioethical interest.[3] At a minimum, it would suggest some unfinished business left over from the supposed victory of patient autonomy over paternalism.

The history of "patient-centered care" over the past three decades suggests three distinct phases. First the concept was employed as medical epistemology, to better characterize the ideal diagnostic process, and in turn, to better organize and guide medical pedagogy. Next the concept became a goal or means of medical therapy. Finally, the concept is being used as a broad framework for policy and health-care organization.

## :: Phase One: Epistemology

In 1977, George Engel, an internist working in the department of psychiatry at the University of Rochester, published a paper that exerted considerable influence over medical educators, especially those involved in training primary-care physicians. Engel proposed a "biopsychosocial model" as an antidote to medicine's increasing biological and molecular reductionism, arguing that the disciplines of psychology and the social sciences were as pertinent to medical research and practice as were the traditional basic biological sciences usually taught in the medical curriculum.[4]

Engel's model was congruent with work already underway at the Department of Family Medicine at the University of Western Ontario, whose chair, Ian McWhinney, is one of the most philosophically well-read leaders of academic family medicine. McWhinney had for a long time been interested in the initial, "real" reasons patients came to see the doctor, as distinct from the diagnoses made by the physician at the conclusion of the encounter. Among the younger faculty he recruited to his department were many whose major interest was in quantitative research and educational assessment. They insisted that anything that was taught to their residents about the physician–patient relationship ought to be subjected to careful measurement, both so that it could be taught, and so that the success of the teaching could be assessed.

Dr. Joseph Levenstein, a general practitioner from South Africa, spent 1981–1982 as a visiting professor in McWhinney's department. He had independently been trying to answer a question asked him by a medical student—what method did he employ that allowed him to use his prior knowledge of the personality and social context of his patients to provide them with more effective medical care? Levenstein began audiotaping and analyzing his interviews and developing a typology to rank them from most to least effective. Levenstein, along with McWhinney's group, eventually organized their joint insights into their "patient-centered clinical method."[5] As they formulated this method, they recognized similarities to the observations of the pioneering British psychiatrist Michael Balint, and to Carl Rogers's concept of client-centered counseling.[6]

As first proposed, the "patient-centered clinical method" called for the physician to engage in two parallel tracks of inquiry. Along one track, the physician needed to do the traditional medical work of gathering a history, conducting a physical exam along with appropriate laboratory and imaging studies, and reaching a diagnosis. The other track consisted of eliciting the patient's experience of the episode of illness, along with whatever practical consequences the illness and the fear of potential outcomes posed for the patient's life. The physician's work was not complete until some accommodation had been reached between the two tracks. Making an accurate diagnosis and recommending proper treatment were insufficient, if the patient's concerns, feelings, and issues had not been satisfactorily addressed as well. The Western Ontario group continued to expand and refine this model, primarily with the goals of conducting research on its effectiveness and of breaking it down into teachable elements for their trainees.[7]

In 1994, a task force funded by the Pew Memorial Trust and the Fetzer Foundation produced a report on "relationship-centered care."

The intended audience was educators of health professionals, who were admonished to keep always in mind the need to key their educational efforts to three relationships: that between health professional and patient; that among the different health professionals; and that among the patient, health professional, and community.[8] Since "patient-centered care" appears from the first to have assumed a physician–patient relationship, for our purposes, patient-centered care and relationship-centered care may be viewed as synonymous. The basic motivation for both appears to be the same—a dissatisfaction with reductionistic biomedical models of "science" as the basis for medical education and practice.

## ▪▪ Phase Two: Therapy

The clinical scientists at Western Ontario had little interest in teaching their residents a method of interacting with patients, if they could not demonstrate that this method would lead to enhanced clinical outcomes. Following earlier work by Starfield, the Western Ontario physicians, led by Martin Bass, showed that patients treated according to the patient-centered approach showed enhanced relief of symptoms, in some cases long after the initial encounter.[9] The studies suggested that the patient-centered method did not lead to improved outcomes by helping the physician to make a more accurate diagnosis, and then ordering more appropriate tests or therapies; rather, patient-centeredness appeared to have an independent therapeutic effect.

The therapeutic benefits of listening more carefully to patients, and making them feel as if they are active partners in the medical care process, have now been shown in a number of research trials and meta-analyses.[10] Perhaps the most striking demonstration came from the Medical Outcomes Study, where investigators showed that the more participatory approach to patients improved the outcomes of a number of common chronic illnesses.[11]

## ▪▪ Phase Three: Policy and the Medical Home

We can fast-forward this account to a report published in 2004 as a result of the work of seven national family medicine organizations, called "The Future of Family Medicine."[12] At the turn of the twenty-first century, the specialty of family medicine was in crisis. The numbers of U.S. medical school graduates choosing that specialty were declining, due both to lower income levels compared to other specialties, and to perceptions of a heavy workload, long hours on call, and pressures from managed care insurance to move patients through quickly in assembly-line fashion. The organizations began by conducting extensive focus-group research to find out what American patients thought family medicine was or should be, and what they were looking for in the physician and the office staff and setting.

The final report compiled by the family medicine panel appealed to two central, interrelated themes—"patient-centered care" and the "personal medical home."[13] The model proposed for patient-centered care incorporated but went beyond the initial work at Western Ontario. The report characterized these two concepts as follows:

> *Patient-centered care:*…based on a physician–patient relationship that is highly satisfying and humanizing to the patient and the physician (as well as other practice clinicians)…the patient, not the physician, occupies center stage. From first contact through the completion of the care episode, the patient must meet with consistent and competent care…all patients will receive care that is culturally and linguistically appropriate…practices strive to meet patient and community needs for integrated care by giving patients what they want and need—preventive care, acute care, rehabilitative care, chronic illness care, and supportive care—when they want and need it by anticipating patient needs and by designing services to meet those needs.[14]

> *Personal medical home:*…steps must be taken to ensure that every American has a personal medical home that serves as the focal point through which all individuals—regardless of age, sex, race, or socioeconomic status—receive a basket of acute, chronic, and preventive medical care services. Through their medical home, patients can be assured of care that is not only accessible but also accountable, comprehensive, integrated, patient-centered, safe, scientifically valid, and satisfying to both patients and their physicians.[15]

It seems clear from these statements that the family medicine leaders intended, via the twin concepts, to incorporate a number of contemporary "movements" into the "future of family medicine":

- A medical consumer-rights movement
- The evidence-based medicine movement
- The movement toward increased use of electronic health records
- The patient safety and error-reduction movement

- The movement toward culturally sensitive care
- Health reform and universal access to health care

A final point worth noting is that the authors of the report clearly believe that patient-centered care delivered within a personal medical home will be much more satisfying than the present medical system *for both patient and physician.* The concepts are at least in part a recruitment tool designed to convince graduating medical students that a future career in family medicine can be emotionally satisfying and fulfilling.

The two concepts are beginning to attract wider attention. For example, Karen Davis and her colleagues at the Commonwealth Fund addressed early in 2007 the policy options for "slowing the growth of U.S. health care expenditures," to remove one of the key barriers to affordable health insurance for all. One of six major options they discussed was "changing the health system to promote patient-centered primary care." They cited research showing that the costs of care in different regions of the United States was inversely related to the percentage of medical practitioners from primary care specialties, while quality of care in high-primary-care regions was either equal to or slightly better than elsewhere.[16] They also noted with approval that all three primary care specialty societies (internal medicine, pediatrics, and family medicine) had endorsed the medical home concept, and that the Tax Relief and Health Care Act of 2006 included provisions for a Medicare Medical Home Demonstration Project, with special management fees and incentive payments for physicians who offered medical-home-type coordination of services.[17]

## :: Practical Policy Applications

In what way would the medical practice designed to adhere to the ideals of patient-centered care and the medical home differ from the model most commonly seen today? I here return to the "Future of Family Medicine" report, which lays out a number of practical implications of these concepts.

Some aspects of the redesigned medical practice would be largely out of sight for the patient. The model envisions increased use of multidisciplinary teams of health professionals and of computerized medical records and information systems. The electronic record, in turn, would be employed as a vehicle to enhance error reduction and increase patient safety.

In other ways, however, the new practice design would be highly visible to the patient:

- *Improved access:* the new practice would employ strategies for enhanced scheduling of visits, including same-day scheduling for most medical needs. Hours would be expanded to improve patient convenience. Patients would be offered several options, including e-mail, Internet access to lab results, and so on, for communicating with their physicians and office staff.
- *Redesigned office:* The traditional waiting room would disappear, to be replaced by a patient health resource center. Larger rooms would accommodate group visits, where a dozen or so patients with common chronic conditions, like diabetes, could all be seen at the same time, facilitating patient education while enhancing social support and mutual advice-sharing among the patients.
- *Expanded service:* through the use of a multidisciplinary team, emphasis would be placed on offering an increased array of services directly through the office. Referrals to other facilities for services not available in the office would still occur, with the office taking more responsibility for coordinating and integrating those services into the ongoing care of the patient, ideally utilizing the electronic health record as a tool.[18]
- *Patient/community advisory board:* This strategy is not explicitly addressed in the "Future of Family Medicine," but seems consistent with its major themes, especially with the announced goal of "care provided within a community context."[19] It is standard for a federally qualified community health center—the sort of practice that today may come closest to realizing the full potential of the proposed model—to include a community advisory board in its administrative structure. It would seem logical that all "medical homes" would wish to include a representative panel of patients and family members from the community to assist in the development of practice policies.

In summary, it appears that the "patient-centered medical home" goes well beyond simply putting up new wallpaper. Both the conduct of daily activities in the office, and the general "feel" of the patient's experience there, will be quite different.[20] These changes at least hold out promise that the needs and values of the patient will become much more powerful drivers of the staff's activities than is now all too often the case.[21]

I find it striking that a group of physicians should have been contemplating changes in the basic structure of medical care in the United States, in a direction that seems to offer important *practical* enhancements in patient autonomy, with so little input or even attention from bioethicists.


## ⠶ Accept No Imitations

In recent years, two other "movements" have gained ground, which superficially might suggest important resemblances to patient-centered care. On further analysis, they appear actually to be quite different.

Scientists at the National Institutes of Health and in academic medicine generally have recently begun to tout the virtues of "personalized medicine." While such a term might mean many things, its overriding focus appears to be the promise of the new genomic science. The argument is that, once we understand the human genome, we need never give (for example) a drug to a patient that will cause an untoward side effect. Before administering the drug, we will do a study of the patient's genome and discover that this patient carries the gene responsible for that adverse drug reaction, so we will prescribe a different drug that does not have these dangers. By knowing the genome, we can precisely tailor medical interventions, both diagnostic and therapeutic, to the individual patient.[22]

Personalized medicine, in this view, might be a great advance. But it would not escape from the reductionist biomedical model that was the core reason why patient-entered care was seen as a necessary alternative. According to this view, we are our DNA. To treat us *as a unique person* is simply to know our gene sequences. Such a formula seems inadequate for a truly patient-centered medicine.

The other look-alike is "boutique" medicine. Many physicians have become disgusted with the content and the tempo of the mass-produced patient encounter that appears to them to be dictated by today's reimbursement system—what might be called "Hamstercare," using the metaphor of a hamster running ever faster inside a wire wheel in a cage.[23] Some have rebelled by cutting their patient lists to roughly a quarter of their previous patient load, promising a variety of personalized services such as home visits, longer visit times, and around-the-clock availability, and charging a surcharge of perhaps $5000 per year beyond insurance reimbursement of payments for specific services.[24]

The forces at work in modern medicine that have prompted some physicians to see the need for fundamental reform and therefore to embrace the patient-centered "cause" appear to be in large part the same forces that have promoted the appearance of boutique medicine. In each case, it is argued that physician and patient satisfaction will increase simultaneously. But it is important to remember that patient-centered medicine assumes a commitment to assuring access to the community of patients. It is not consistent with disenfranchising three-fourths of the community in order to offer five-star medical care to the remaining high bidders. Patient-centered care includes an element of justice that is lacking in boutique medicine.[25]

## ⠃ Generosity and Joy?

The "Future of Family Medicine" describes the model practice as "people taking care of people."[26] We have already noted the expressed hope that it will not only be the case that patients will be happier in this new setting, but also that physicians and staff will be happier, and that this will help to reverse the flight of graduating medical students away from careers in primary care.

Sociologist Arthur Frank's book, *The Renewal of Generosity,* was published in the same year that the "Future of Family Medicine" report appeared.[27] Otherwise, one might have concluded all the more rapidly that Frank had simply gone off the deep end. Frank is not content with calling for a return of a sense of generosity to the relationship between physician and patient. He even goes as far as to insist upon *joy:*

> Beyond learning from others, suffering with others, entering a boundary space between me and the other, is there joy in the presence of others? Do I feel pleasure in their presence, and do they seem pleased to be with me? Am I putting up with my fellow humans, as Marcus [Aurelius] too often seems to be; do I feel nothing more than responsibility for them, which seems a limit for Levinas? What lies beyond Marcus and Levinas is promised by Anatole Broyard's wonderful phrase: that he sought a place where he and his physician could *frolic* together. What have I done, today, to increase the time and space of frolic? We need more stories of frolic; I regret I have offered so few. I hear so few.[28]

Frank's mention of "joy" in this strange context reminded me of one other time that I had heard the word used. Around 1985, faculty at the College of Human Medicine, Michigan State University, gathered to design a major curriculum overhaul. A senior pediatrician, the late Ray Helfer, chastised the group for the somber tone of much of the deliberations.

Where, he asked, was the *joy* of learning medicine? There was an embarrassed silence. I attributed the embarrassment to two sources. Some of those present, I imagined, felt the import of Helfer's criticism and were chagrined that we had not done better in his estimation. Others, I suspected, were embarrassed that a highly respected faculty member had injected into the meeting such an obviously irrelevant comment.

Let us grant for a moment that "joy" may be a bit over the top. People do not want to get cancer just so that they will have an excuse to frolic with the urologist. Many people encountering today's health-care system, such as Sylvia Stultz, would be immensely grateful just for a little bit of basic civility, never mind joy. So let us ratchet down expectations and ask what it might take for people to feel *welcomed* by their doctors and other caregivers. This is the likely intersection between Frank's call for generosity in medicine and the notion of the medical home. The point about *going home* is that one expects to be welcomed, to be treated with a level of generosity based simply on who one is—that one is a member of the family—not on what one has done lately for anyone else, or how much one can afford to pay. Laurie Zoloth, who like Frank is inspired by the philosophy of Emanuel Levinas, might view the medical home as a way to focus our notion of *hospitality*—to ask, what is the medical equivalent of the tent of Abraham and Sarah, situated at the crossroads, with open sides, lit at night with fires that could be seen for miles, where any wayfarer would be welcomed?[29]

Is it a role for the bioethicist to watch carefully the development of the "medical home" concept, to help to assure that we do not lose sight of this basic human need to be *welcomed* when the fates have beaten us up a bit? For all the good intentions of patient-centered care and the medical home, it may be too easy to become overly focused on which electronic-health-record program works best, or on how to get properly reimbursed for group meetings for diabetic care and education. What has to happen in a medical office so that patients feel welcomed on arrival and throughout the visit?[30] What sorts of care do the staff need so that they can go on, day after day, being welcoming to people, while still doing all the other things that need to be done?[31]

## ⠺ A Patient-Centered Bioethics

Supposing that the interview between Sylvia Stultz and the surgical oncologist had raised an "interesting" ethical question. Perhaps there were two possible surgical approaches to the tumor, one potentially more mutilating but with much better survival odds, and Ms. Stultz had refused that surgery for reasons the oncologist thought irrational. How would this "ethics case" be presented to us in a textbook or journal article? In all likelihood the "case" would look little different from the standard medical case write-up, starting with the "presentation" of the patient to the physician—that is, whatever happened in the exam or consultation room starting at 3:30 P.M. Being inured as we are to medical jargon, we probably would not even notice that the same word had been used for the arrival of the sick person as is used to describe how an upscale restaurant arranges the food on the plate for maximum esthetic effect.

From Ms. Stultz's point of view, when did her story as a patient begin? It might have been at 10:15 that morning when she actually entered the waiting room, only to be forced to sit for more than five hours. Or it might have begun whenever she first detected some sign from her body that things were not as they had usually been in the past.

Medical anthropologists sometimes speak of the "lay referral system" to designate the social processes by which an individual comes, first, to define himself as being ill rather than well, and second, to seek the help of any particular caregiver, either traditional healer or licensed practitioner. The concept is useful for reminding physicians (and bioethicists) that a lot of decisions have to be made, most of them on "nonmedical" grounds, before the medical encounter itself begins. A medicocentric world view that assumes that the start of the encounter is the start of everything interesting and worth recording or observing is therefore deeply flawed.[32]

When exactly the story of a bioethics "case" properly begins, of course, is just one of many features of how we carry out the activities that are ascribed to our field. I use it here merely to illustrate how, despite the supposed triumph of patient autonomy, bioethics still adheres to a medically dominated rather than a patient-focused worldview.[33]

I believe that most physicians who have seriously confronted the possibility that being "patient-centered" requires opening and closing our office when the patients wish to be seen, and not when we and our staff prefer to work, experienced a modest epiphany, an "aha!" moment. Taking the patient-centered-care movement seriously might lead to bioethics's having its own "aha!" moment, or a series of them, about ways in which the patient's point of view still remains opaque to us, despite our many well-intentioned efforts at both the theoretical and practical levels. If one of our objectives as a field is that the voice of the patient ought to be clearly heard whenever health-care decisions are being made, then it seems we have considerably more work to do. In order to accomplish that task, bioethics needs to forge a closer alliance with primary care medicine.

NOTES TO CHAPTER 3

1. Okie S. Teaching hospitals how to listen: one woman struggled to convince administrators that staff responsiveness—or lack of it—affects patient outcomes. *Washington Post*, December 12, 2006:HE1.
2. Lindemann H. Bioethics' gender. *Am J Bioethics* 6(2):W15–W19, 2006.
3. We will see, in our historical account to follow, that the years during which patient-centered care was gaining ground in medical thinking overlapped with the early days of the "patient autonomy movement" in bioethics. One might claim that, had bioethics not prepared the ground by focusing attention on the value of respecting patient autonomy, the seeds of patient-centered care might not have sprouted. This argument posits a connection between bioethics and patient-centered care. It does not explain why bioethicists, as a group, have paid so little attention to the latter concept.
4. Engel GL. The need for a new medical model: a challenge to biomedicine. *Science* 196:129–36, 1977; see also Engel GL. How long must medicine's science be bound by a seventeenth century world view? In: White KL (ed.). *The task of medicine: dialogue at Wickenberg*. Menlo Park, CA: Henry J. Kaiser Family Foundation, 1988, pp. 113–36.
5. Levenstein JH, McCracken EC, McWhinney IR, et al. The patient-centered clinical method. 1. A model for the doctor-patient interaction in family medicine. *Fam Pract* 3:24–30, 1986.
6. Balint M. *The doctor, the patient, and his illness*. New York: International Universities Press, 1957; Rogers C. *Client-centered therapy: its current practice implications and theory*. Cambridge, MA: Riverside, 1951.
7. Stewart M, Brown JB, Weston WW, et al. *Patient-centered medicine: transforming the clinical method*. Thousand Oaks, CA: Sage Publications, 1995. In turn, credit is given to Pendleton D, Schofield T, Tate P, Havelock P. *The consultation: an approach to learning and teaching*. Oxford: Oxford University Press, 1984.
8. Tresolini CP, Pew-Fetzer Task Force. *Health professions education and relationship-centered care*. San Francisco, CA: Pew Health Professions Commission, 1994.
9. Bass MJ, Buck C, Turner L, et al. The physician's actions and the outcome of illness in family practice. *J Fam Pract* 23:43–47, 1986; Bass BJ, McWhinney IR, Dempsey JB, et al. Predictors of outcomes in headache patients presenting to family physicians–a one year prospective study. *Headache J* 26:285–94, 1986; Starfield B, Wray C, Hess K, et al. The influence of patient-practitioner agreement on outcome of care. *Am J Publ Health* 71:127–32, 1981.

10. Bodenheimer T, Wagner EH, Grumbach K. Improving primary care for patients with chronic illness. *JAMA* 288:1775–9, 2002.
11. Kaplan SH, Greenfield S, Ware JE. Assessing the effects of physician-patient interactions on the outcome of chronic disease. *Med Care* 27: S110–S127, 1989.
12. Martin JC, Avant RF, Bowman MA, et al. The future of family medicine: a collaborative project of the family medicine community. *Ann Fam Med* 2 (Suppl 1):S3–S32, 2004.
13. In proposing the "personal medical home" model, the family medicine group credited the prior work of the American Academy of Pediatrics. The notion of a "medical home" originated among pediatricians concerned about the coordinated care of children with special needs, such as those with cerebral palsy. The first recorded use of the term "medical home" was in a handbook prepared in 1967; Sia C, Tonniges TF, Osterhus E, Taba S. History of the medical home concept. *Pediatrics* 113 (5 suppl):1473–8, 2004. More recently, the American College of Physicians has also endorsed the "medical home" concept; American College of Physicians. *The advanced medical home: a patient-centered, physician-guided model of health care.* Philadelphia: American College of Physicians, January 30, 2006; http://www.acponline.org/hpp/adv_med.pdf (accessed January 30, 2007).
14. Martin JC, Avant RF, Bowman MA, et al. The future of family medicine: a collaborative project of the family medicine community. *Ann Fam Med* 2 (Suppl 1):S3–S32, 2004, quote on p. S14.
15. Martin JC, Avant RF, Bowman MA, et al. The future of family medicine: a collaborative project of the family medicine community, quote on p. S14, footnote omitted.
16. Fisher ES, Wennberg DE, Stukel TA, et al. The implications of regional variations in Medicare spending. Part 1: The content, quality, and accessibility of care. *Ann Intern Med* 138:273–87, 2003; Fisher ES, Wennberg DE, Stukel TA, et al. The implications of regional variations in Medicare spending. Part 2: Health outcomes and satisfaction with care. *Ann Intern Med* 138:288–98, 2003.
17. Davis K, Schoen C, Guterman S, et al. *Slowing the growth of U.S. health care expenditures: what are the options?* New York: The Commonwealth Fund, January, 2007, pp. 12, 22–3, http://www.cmwf.org/usr_doc/Davis_slowing growthUShltcareexpenditureswhatareoptions_989.pdf (accessed February 1, 2007).
18. Martin JC, Avant RF, Bowman MA, et al. The future of family medicine: a collaborative project of the family medicine community, pp. S3–S32, esp. pp. S13–S17.
19. Martin JC, Avant RF, Bowman MA, et al. The future of family medicine: a collaborative project of the family medicine community, quote on p. S14.
20. The Commonwealth Fund 2003 National Survey of Physicians and the Quality of Care indicated that one-fourth of U.S. primary care physicians currently incorporate major elements of patient-centered care in their

practices: Davis K, Schoenbaum SC, Audet AM. A 2020 vision of patient-centered primary care. *J Gen Intern Med* 20:953–7, 2005.

21. Since a limited or conservative view does not appear to be a criticism that one could offer on the "Future of Family Medicine" report, the opposite concern has been raised—how such an enhanced and expanded office will be viable financially, absent wholesale reform of the U.S. health care system, which the family medicine experts did not foresee in the near future. A financial model was proposed to suggest that the model was realistic as long as some relatively minor changes in reimbursement were forthcoming: Spann SJ, Task Force 6 and the Executive Editorial Team. Report on financing the new model of family medicine. *Ann Fam Med* 2 (Suppl 3):S1–S21, 2004. For example, it would probably be necessary that primary care physicians be fairly reimbursed for time spent on e-mail contacts with patients and for group visits, both of which are currently difficult to achieve, given the insurance system's fixation on a face-to-face encounter between a physician and a single patient. A good deal of the financial viability of the "new" medical office hinges on predictions of cost savings related to full implementation of electronic records.

22. Abrahams E, Ginsburg GS, Silver M. The Personalized Medicine Coalition: goals and strategies. *Am J Pharmacogenomics* 5:345–55, 2005.

23. Morrison I . *Health care in the new millennium: visions, values, and leadership.* San Francisco: Jossey-Bass, 2000:27–8. Morrison uses the hamster-in-a-cage analogy but does not actually use the term "HamsterCare" so far as I can see; I believe that this final turn of phrase is the contribution of academic family physician Joseph Scherger.

24. Alexander GC, Kurlander J, Wynia MK. Physicians in retainer ("concierge") practice: A national survey of physician, patient, and practice characteristics. *J Gen Intern Med* 20:1079–83, 2005.

25. Charatan F. US "boutique medicine" could threaten care for the majority. *BMJ* 324:187, 2002; Jones JW, McCullough LB, Richman BW. Ethics of boutique medical practice. *J Vasc Surg* 39:1354–5, 2004. One of the best existing models for the primary care "medical home" is the federally qualified community health center, which is designed especially for the care of financially disadvantaged populations, and so is about as far removed from boutique medicine as one can get.

26. Martin JC, Avant RF, Bowman MA, et al. The future of family medicine: a collaborative project of the family medicine community. *Ann Fam Med* 2 (Suppl 1): S3–S32, 2004, quote on p. S14.

27. Frank AW. *The renewal of generosity: illness, medicine, and how to live.* Chicago: University of Chicago Press, 2004.

28. Frank AW. *The renewal of generosity: illness, medicine, and how to live,* p. 142. The reference (omitted) is to Broyard A. *Intoxicated by my illness.* New York: Clarkson Potter, 1992, p. 45. Frank actually misquotes Broyard slightly. Broyard says, "While he inevitably feels superior to me because he is the doctor and I am the patient, I'd like him to know that I feel superior to him, too, that he is my patient also and I have my diagnosis of

him. There should be a place where *our respective superiorities* could meet and frolic together" [emphasis added].

29. Zoloth L. I want you: notes toward a theory of hospitality. In: Eckenwiler LA, Cohn FG, eds. *The ethics of bioethics: mapping the moral landscape.* Baltimore: Johns Hopkins University Press, 2007, pp. 205–19.

30. An interesting experiment, being tried in some primary-care offices, is to assign a single staff member to each patient on arrival. Instead of being handed off from receptionist to nursing assistant to physician, and so on, the patient remains with this staff person from beginning to end, so that all transitions flow smoothly. (During the physician visit, for instance, the staff member becomes the secretary, completing the medical record notes.) Reportedly this method greatly increases patient satisfaction and office efficiency; whether it is cost-effective has yet to be determined. See, for example, the "Care by Design" project at the University of Utah Department of Family Medicine, http://healthcare.utah.edu/ publicaffairs/spotlight/spotlight_461.html (accessed December 29, 2007).

31. In *The Healer's Power,* I described this basic tension as that of "care versus work"; Brody H. *The healer's power.* New Haven, CT: Yale University Press, 1992, pp. 66–82.

32. Similarly corrective to a medicocentric view are studies of the occurrence of symptoms in the general population, showing that at any given time, there are many more people who experience backache (for example) than ever seek medical care for their symptoms. A classic description of this phenomenon is Hannay DR. *The symptom iceberg: a study of community health.* Boston: Routledge and Kegan Paul, 1979.

33. For this point I am most grateful to my former colleagues in the Center for Ethics and Humanities in the Life Sciences, Michigan State University. For some years we discussed writing a series of papers called "the view from the bed," to try to envision what a properly patient-centered approach to bioethical issues would actually look like. The project never came to fruition. Several bioethicists have produced works intended for a popular audience, but these books tend to resemble medical self-help or advice books and do not necessarily shift one's gaze substantially from a medical viewpoint; see, for example, Radey C. *Choosing wisely: how patients and their families can make the right decisions about life and death.* New York: Doubleday/Image, 1992.

# 4 ⠶

# Evidence-Based Medicine and
# Pay-for-Performance

Over roughly the past fifteen years, there has been a revolution in how both academic physicians and medical practitioners view medical knowledge. This in turn has led to a revolution in how physicians and hospitals are reimbursed. Both revolutions have considerable potential to alter the face of medicine and how it treats patients.

If one were to peruse the bioethics literature during this period, one would have to conclude that neither revolution occurred. When I began working on the project that has led to this book, I did a PubMed search on "ethics" and "pay-for-performance" and retrieved no articles.[1] Bioethics, during this time, has remained occupied with old issues, such as controversial aspects of end-of-life care, and new issues, such as neuroethics and nanotechnology. Why bioethics has found evidence-based medicine (EBM) and pay-for-performance (P4P) so unworthy of its attention should give us pause. I will offer some hypotheses at the end of the chapter.

First, some definitions. EBM advocates have offered several formal definitions.[2] For our purposes we can distill from these formal definitions two key proposals of EBM—first, that clinical decisions ought to be based on the available evidence of the highest methodological quality; and second, that those who appeal to the body of evidence ought to be very explicit in assessing the quality of the evidence that is being used.[3] (It is worth noting that one can employ either criterion of EBM independently of the other.) Accompanying the first criterion is, usually, a hierarchical listing of types of research studies, in which it is claimed that randomized controlled trials (RCTs) and meta-analyses of RCTs occupy the highest rung of the evidence ladder.

P4P is an attempt to address a basic paradox of the financing of medical care. Previously, no one had yet developed a reimbursement system that would pay the physician when, and only when, she does something that benefits the patient. The fee-for-service system rewards physicians for doing unnecessary things, and capitated managed care rewarded physicians for omitting necessary things. Paying physicians on straight salary rewards them for going home promptly at five.

The advent of EBM seemed to offer a breakthrough. Using EBM methods we could decide what interventions really benefited patients. We could then watch physicians carefully and pay them when they performed those interventions. Or, even better, we could measure the health status of the patients and pay physicians depending on the actual health outcomes that they achieved.

To go from EBM to P4P therefore requires at least the following steps:

- Assessing the medical literature based on methodological quality of evidence
- Developing practice guidelines utilizing the highest-quality evidence
- Developing measuring tools to determine how well practitioners and hospitals adhere to the practice-based guidelines
- Developing reimbursement structures selectively to reward guideline adherence

Two different levels of P4P can be distinguished. Often, the measurements needed to implement a P4P system work well only when there is a critical mass of patients or of clinical services. A certain number of bad health outcomes are due simply to bad luck, and studying small numbers of patients risks over-counting results that physicians really cannot control. So proposals to implement P4P in the reimbursement provided to hospitals or to large physician practice groups have sometimes been favored over schemes by which individual physicians would be reimbursed according to a P4P formula. I believe that P4P applied to individual physicians, or small physician groups, is most ethically problematic, so I will focus especially on that level of proposal.

The position that I defend is generally pro-EBM and anti-P4P. On balance (perhaps because, as I will discuss below, EBM represents a net power shift within medicine toward my own academic colleagues in primary care), I believe that the EBM movement has been helpful, and has served to correct a number of unfortunate tendencies. It seems reasonable to claim that EBM has relatively little to fear from its enemies, whose criticisms are often off the mark, and more to fear from its friends, especially those who make inflated claims for it.[4] P4P, by contrast, while quite attractive in theory, seems to have emerged as a recommended practical strategy far in advance of any convincing evidence that it accomplishes what it is supposed to do. In short, for the foreseeable future, P4P is not evidence-based. Finally, I will ask what implications P4P as a general concept has for professionalism in medicine.

## ∷ Rival Narratives and a Medical Power Shift

Laypersons, on being told for the first time that there is a new movement called EBM, naturally wonder what in heaven's name the old medicine was based on, if not evidence—and scientific evidence at that. For all the rhetoric that EBM has generated, it seems clear that the pre-EBM practice of medicine was strongly "evidence-based" in some sense. The EBM rhetoric tends to hide the fact that a major shift occurred in what was seen to count as "the best" evidence within the world of academic medicine. This shift amounted to a major power grab by one subset of academic physicians—a point that few medical historians and social scientists appear to have appreciated so far.[5] We can best grasp how one group wrested power from the other if we analyze two narratives of medical knowledge that have been especially favored by the two camps.

For many years, whenever one wished to defend the power of the medical-academic status quo, one trotted out the story told by Lewis Thomas, a distinguished pathologist and cancer researcher, in his popular column in the *New England Journal of Medicine*.[6] Thomas told the story of how, in the 1940s, the most advanced form of medical technology available to treat victims of polio was the iron lung, a primitive form of respirator that worked by cyclically changing the pressure applied to the outside of the chest wall. Thousands of these machines were found in the wards of U.S. hospitals during and after polio epidemics, and many lives were saved by them.

Then came the identification of the precise viruses that cause polio, and the development of vaccines against those viruses—first the Salk or killed-virus vaccine, and later the Sabin live, attenuated virus vaccine. In a few years, these iron lungs could no longer be seen in hospital wards, and presumably were then gathering rust in a junkyard.[7]

According to Thomas, the iron lung was a prototypical example of what he termed "halfway technology." It could have some ameliorating effect on the course of the disease, but could not cure or eliminate it. The actual eradication of polio depended on real technology, the vaccine. Real technology, in turn, required a full understanding of the disease process at the cellular or molecular level. Thomas went on to claim that the vast majority of medical treatments then in use were halfway technologies; so the field was wide open for medicine to be transformed by the next generation of Salks and Sabins. We would discover, for example, that juvenile diabetes was caused by a virus that attacked and destroyed the islet cells in the pancreas, or perhaps through an interacting set of dysfunctional genes. As soon as we had developed the ideal vaccine or method of gene replacement therapy, we could throw the old halfway technology, insulin injections, out the window. Moreover, the replacement of halfway technology with real technology was bound to save money, just as the expensive iron lung was supplanted by a dose of vaccine that cost pennies.

Thomas's polio narrative and the term "halfway technology" were widely quoted by defenders of the most powerful clique within academic medicine. These consisted, first, of basic scientists who performed traditional bench research in the laboratory; and their clinical colleagues, medical subspecialists who focused their attention on a very narrow range of diseases so that they could best understand the basic mechanisms of the disease process. The smugness with which the polio story was retold failed to take into account the difficulty of finding any new stories, besides polio, of the replacement of halfway technology with real technology, let alone any case in which the new technology actually saved anyone any money.

Today, when EBM advocates gather around the pot-bellied stove in the general store and swap stories, they usually begin with the encainide-flecainide or Cardiac Arrhythmia Suppression Trial (CAST) story.[8] In the late 1980s there were several things that everyone knew. One of the major causes of death following a heart attack was abnormal heart rhythms. These abnormal rhythm patterns could, in turn, be reduced significantly by giving certain drugs, and such drugs were routinely used in heart attack victims. The electrophysiology of these abnormal rhythms, and the pharmacology of the drugs that suppressed them, were both well understood.

It would appear utterly superfluous, given what was then known, to do an actual clinical trial of the value of arrhythmia suppression after heart attack. But it became valuable to know which of two rival drugs, encainide or flecainide, did a better job of suppressing these nasty rhythms, and some busybody went on to insist that this trial ought to have a placebo control group. (According to the doctrine of "clinical equipoise" to guide the ethics of human subjects research, the placebo control group would have been deemed unethical; but the paper by Benjamin Freedman that represented the classic statement of clinical equipoise was published only after the CAST trial, in all probability, had been planned.[9])

When the CAST trialists reported their preliminary results in the *New England Journal*, they turned "what everybody knew" upside down. The trial had to be discontinued early because of excess deaths in the groups receiving encainide and flecainide. What "everyone knows," today, is that drugs of this general class cause more harm than allowing the arrhythmias to continue. Heart-attack victims still die of fatal arrhythmias, but the "cure" of drug treatment turns out to be worse than the disease.

The moral that the EBM advocates draw from the CAST tale is that no matter how well one understands the cellular and molecular phenomena associated with any disease or therapy, one cannot know what will actually happen in human patients in community settings until one studies those outcomes in those patients. The powerful leaders of academic medicine in the old era had assumed that once one possessed that basic level of knowledge, it would be simple to extrapolate that knowledge to the intact human organism, and from the research laboratory to the ambulatory setting. What CAST showed—and what was eventually shown by a large number of similar trials—is that such extrapolations were very far from being slam-dunks.

If subspecialized bench research now turns out to be second-class knowledge, whereas clinical trials that measure outcomes of real interest (like death rates) in real patients are the new gold standard, then the old guard in academic medicine must stand aside to allow a new elite to take over.[10] The basic scientists of the new elite were the clinical epidemiologists and biostatisticians who best understood RCT methodology. The clinicians of the new elite were the primary-care physicians who had ready access to "real" patients in community settings and who could assess which trial outcomes were most pertinent to an individual's life and health. The old guard of academic medicine had managed to hang onto power, despite numerous challenges, throughout the "post-Flexnerian" period of the twentieth century.[11] How the new EBM elite managed to wrest power from them is a fascinating historical tale that has yet to be fully told.

This power shift in academic medicine would be of no interest to bioethics were it not for what it signaled about medical epistemology. The power shift was made possible by a redefinition of what counted as *the best evidence*. Medical practice pre-EBM was very strongly evidence-based, but the "evidence" referred to events that occurred at the lowest levels of the hierarchy of natural systems in a biopsychosocial model—at the level of cells and molecules.[12] By contrast, what counted as "good evidence" in the new EBM world tended to cluster at the middle and sometimes the higher levels of this systems hierarchy, more commonly involving the intact human organism and human populations.

The power shift obscured the fact that each appeal to evidence was a part of medicine's age-old effort to vanquish uncertainty. Kathryn Montgomery, in a book that features one of the most sophisticated treatments of EBM, notes that uncertainty can never be eliminated from medicine, which is at its root a practical craft (not a science) that attempts to apply scientific knowledge to individual cases.[13] An anecdote that seems to capture the core of Montgomery's message is:

> Renowned for breeding lions in captivity, [a Dublin] zookeeper was asked the secret of his success.
> "You must understand lions," he said.
> "What is it that you have to know about lions?" the interviewer asked.
> "Ah, well," said the zookeeper, "you need to understand: every lion is different."[14]

In other words, whenever a group of medical scientists claims that if one would only follow their methods, one could eliminate that pesky uncertainty from medicine for good, something silly is about to happen. We understand better today the silliness of the Lewis Thomas devotees. The question now is whether EBM has any grasp of its own risk of silliness.[15]

## ⠅⠅ Challenges to EBM

One of the difficulties in critiquing EBM is to figure out exactly what one is critiquing. Two very different versions of EBM appear to be abroad in the land, and one could label them "sophisticated" and "crude" EBM, respectively. Sophisticated EBM makes relatively modest claims for itself and agrees that, depending on circumstances, many different forms of evidence might be "the best" evidence. Crude EBM practitioners, by contrast, often make exaggerated claims and generally talk and act as if only one kind of evidence, the RCT, is worth anything at all. While the major books and articles on EBM usually emanate from the sophisticated camp, the form of EBM that physicians in the trenches are most likely to encounter is the crude variety. At times, the sophisticated camp can be disingenuous in providing additional fodder for crude EBM, but then pointing to its own sophistication to deny responsibility.[16]

Some of the critiques launched against EBM, especially from self-styled medical humanists, seem off the mark. For example, it has often been charged that EBM is deleterious to a desired focus on the individual patient because it represents a shift from the individual to the population.[17] Pre-EBM physicians thought about individual patients while EBM physicians think only about population-based data from RCTs.[18] This accusation locates the threat to concern for the individual patient in quite the wrong place. The "traditional" physician who relies mostly on basic science knowledge to guide treatment similarly ignores the individual. He regards this patient, for instance, within the *population* of all those whose heart is on the left side of the chest, or within the *population* of those whose pharyngitis is caused by the streptococcus, even though he is well aware that there are individual exceptions to those supposed rules. For the pre-EBM physician to put on airs about his concern for the individual is much like the pot criticizing the coloration of the kettle.[19] So far as pre-EBM practitioners are concerned, there are no individual human beings walking in the door—only collections of organs, tissues, cells, and molecules.

Turning now to critiques of EBM that have merit, we might first consider the most obvious one. Where is the *evidence* of sufficiently high quality that EBM-based practice produces superior outcomes to traditional practice? Even the strongest advocates of EBM would not be so bold as to claim that such a body of evidence exists, or even that we could conduct the necessary trials to accumulate such evidence.[20] This criticism can probably be dismissed without much discussion. If EBM actually has even a fraction of the various advantages claimed for it, it would be irresponsible to refuse to adopt its tenets until such time as unequivocal evidence supported the transition. If proof of EBM's effectiveness were easy to come by, we might reasonably demand such proof before endorsing EBM methods as general policy. But any such proof would be extremely difficult to attain. Of all the forces and activities that influence physician and health-system behavior and patient outcomes, it would be quite challenging to isolate EBM as a single factor and *prove* that that factor accounted for the positive change. For all we may be able to tell, with EBM included in the mix, things did not get any better; but without EBM, things might have been much worse.

Next, EBM has been attacked for its over-reliance on RCTs. There are many circumstances in which a well-designed observational study provides better and more relevant evidence than does even a well-designed RCT; and there are many other situations where a well-designed observational study will be more reliable than a poorly designed RCT.[21] Here the EBM critic is on firmer ground in arguing that the EBM advocate is ignoring the individual patient. Any RCT represents an *average* effect of trying a treatment on a large number of subjects. Perhaps, overall, drug A significantly outperforms drug B, but there are sure to be individual cases within the subject pool where B outperformed A. If the patient now seeking then physician's care happens to represent those atypical subjects in the most relevant ways, then it would be a mistake to apply the results of the RCT to *this particular* patient. And, in most such cases, we will have no idea what "in the most relevant ways" means.[22]

Sophisticated EBM practitioners have come to recognize this weakness of RCTs by placing at the very top of their evidence hierarchy the "N of 1" RCT.[23] In an N of 1 study, a single patient is given each of the two alternative treatments sequentially in randomized fashion, with both the patient and the physician who judges the outcomes remaining blinded to which treatment is being given at any time. The results of such an RCT would, one supposes, be fully relevant to any idiosyncrasies of that particular patient, and would represent ideally individualized evidence. Of course, N of 1 studies are hardly ever carried out in practice, and for many medical decisions, they would simply be impossible to conduct. So most EBM advocates never do more than nod ceremonially in the direction of the N of 1 trial.

Mark Tonelli has shown that EBM presents its critics with a moving target. When challenged for leaving out an important type of evidence, or some other consideration that seems pertinent to clinical judgment, EBM advocates (at least, the sophisticated ones) respond by inserting this new category of "evidence" into their next published hierarchy of grades of evidence. To cite one example, after being taxed with ignoring patients' preferences for various treatments, EBM supporters now routinely call for the consideration of these preferences. In similar fashion, they have come to admit that physiological theories about how the human body functions, and the physicians' individual clinical experience, both count as "evidence," though of lesser value than RCTs and systematic reviews of RCTs.

Tonelli goes on to argue that these apparent successes of EBM, in expanding its purview to incorporate previously neglected elements, actually expose its fundamental flaws. EBM has discovered no overarching theory or system by which to integrate these disparate elements. Tonelli objects to the rank-ordering in a "hierarchy of evidence" by claiming that some of these sources of information are different in kind and not merely in degree. By saying, in effect, that one should simply place controlled trial evidence, clinical experience, and patient preferences all in a bowl and stir, EBM shows that at core it relies as much on intuition as any of its "unsystematic" opponents.[24]

At a more general level, Maya Goldenberg has assessed EBM from the standpoint of contemporary philosophy of science. She finds EBM to be an odd throwback to logical positivism, a theoretical stance that has steadily lost credibility since the 1960s—although, as we saw Montgomery arguing in Chapter 2, medicine has in that regard remained a sanctuary for logical positivism among the so-called "scientific" fields. Logical positivism held that objective knowledge of the world was possible, and as long as one followed certain rigorous methods of justification, such knowledge would be value-free. Goldenberg states, "EBM's ability to guide healthcare decision-making by appealing to 'the evidence' as the bottom line is attractive to many because it proposes to rationalize this complex social process. Yet it does so through the positivistic elimination of culture, contexts, and the subjects of knowledge production from consideration, a move that permits the use of evidence as a political instrument where power interests can be obscured by seemingly neutral technical resolve."[25] She adds, "The formal methods promoted by EBM to replace so-called 'traditional' medicine's over-reliance on intuition, habits, and unsystematic clinical experience appear to repeat the misplaced effort to separate science from values."[26] Goldenberg concludes, "The appeal to the authority of evidence that characterises evidence-based practice does not *increase* objectivity but rather *obscures* the subjective elements that inescapably enter all forms of human inquiry."[27]

A practical example of how "power interests can be obscured" in EBM is provided by the role of the pharmaceutical industry in the funding and management of RCTs. Numerous cases have occurred in which the industry, and the academic scientists who are the beneficiaries of its grants and other perks, deliberately suppressed the results of RCTs that showed the company's drug in an unfavorable light. Usually this suppression of data becomes known only as a result of unusual circumstances, suggesting that we have as yet become aware only of the tip of the iceberg, and that such data suppression has been much more widespread than we imagine.[28] On average, an industry-funded study is more than four times as likely to show that the drug under study is the superior treatment than are neutrally funded studies.[29] Given that the vast majority of studies of pharmaceuticals today are industry-funded, it does not seem too much of a stretch to say that any system that relies on published RCTs as the major source of evidence upon which to base practice guidelines runs a serious risk of turning control over medical practice over to the pharmaceutical industry.

Finally, bioethicists should be interested in the emergence of a branch of EBM termed "evidence-based ethics." This term was apparently first used by Jon Tyson in 1995, in relation to the intensive care of premature infants.[30] The association of "evidence-based ethics" with the problems of treating neonates with extreme prematurity seems strange. One would imagine that if there was any area of medicine where it was as clear as possible that merely agreeing upon an extensive set of facts would not resolve the outstanding ethical problems, this would be it. On its face, this field of "ethics" would appear to bear out Michael Loughlin's claim that it seems popular today to imagine that one can render any term in medicine more compelling and persuasive by appending the prefix "evidence-based."[31]

According to Pascal Borry and colleagues, "evidence-based ethics" consists of two propositions—first, that ethical decision-making must be based on the best possible medical evidence; and second, that using EBM techniques will assure a higher quality of ethical decision-making. Borry and colleagues proceed to find reasons to doubt the second proposition.[32] Michael Loughlin agrees with their assessment, but wonders why they did not then go on to doubt the first assumption as well. To whom, he wonders, might such a proposition be addressed? Where exactly is the group that is claiming that ethical decisions should be based on outdated or inadequate evidence? "Good ethics depends on good evidence" seems true as long as it remains at the level of platitude. As soon as one moves beyond platitudes, and tries to supply specific criteria for what counts as "the best evidence," one enters controversial territory, and it seems highly arbitrary to attack as "unethical" somebody who judges the quality of the evidence in a different way.[33] Alluding to Hume's classic distinction between "is" and "ought," Loughlin asserts that "evidence-based ethics" is "non-sense"; and adds that the idea that EBM methods would guarantee better ethical decisions must therefore be "non-sense on stilts."[34]

## ∷ P4P: Proposals and Objections

I have argued that it makes little sense to demand that EBM itself produce indisputable evidence for its effectiveness before adopting the sophisticated forms of it as a useful strategy, as long as we add the needed qualifications and understand its limitations. On the other hand, it does seem appropriate to demand that P4P offer some evidence of its practical effectiveness before we endorse its widespread adoption. There are several reasons why this demand seems reasonable. First, in concept, P4P seems hard to argue with; and that is an especially dangerous state of affairs that ought to rouse our suspicions. Second, P4P is likely to be very expensive to implement when we consider the need for impeccable evidence-based practice guidelines, for a method of making the guideline recommendations available to practitioners at the moment that care is being ordered for or delivered to the patient, and for measuring systems to monitor and log what physicians actually do, or fail to do, in all these patient encounters. Third, as we will see, any system for changing physician reimbursement in such a basic way holds potential for considerable collateral damage as well as for improvement.

A little history seems useful here. Prior to P4P, the most significant change in the reimbursement for hospitals was the introduction of the diagnosis-related-group system (DRG) in the mid-1980s. Just as with P4P, DRGs were proposed to eliminate a set of perverse incentives that were driving patient care in the wrong direction. As long as hospitals were paid for each distinct service provided—each day of hospital stay, each drug administered, each x-ray performed—they were clearly given an incentive to do much more for the patient than was actually necessary, and no incentive at all to improve efficiency. The DRG system called for hospitals to be paid by the patient's diagnosis. Once we decided that the average patient with a heart attack could be well cared for at a certain cost, we simply decreed that we would pay that much for each patient whose discharge diagnosis was "heart attack." Some patients would have very bad heart attacks and demand a lot more care; some would have quite limited heart attacks and need much less care; and on average, the hospital ought to do all right. If the hospital invested in improving the efficiency with which it cared for heart-attack patients, it could do better than all right, and pocket the savings as a bonus.

To some extent, the desired goals of DRG reform were obtained, and hospitals addressed efficiency issues with much more enthusiasm after the new payment system was implemented. In other ways, unforeseen consequences seriously limited the hoped-for advantages. A new industry sprang up to feed what came to be called "DRG creep." Consulting firms got rich offering hospitals complex computer programs designed to show how, with the same symptoms, patients could be "up-coded" from a low-reimbursing DRG to a much-higher-paying DRG. Hospitals made more money not by taking better care of patients, or even by becoming more efficient, but by playing the right games with the billing codes. All this was unforeseen, but, in hindsight, easily foreseeable. Any new reimbursement plan is an open invitation to figure out how to game the system.

One of the most impressive studies of P4P in practice, and a study often cited as proof positive that P4P is ready for prime time, illustrates this concern for gaming.[35] Perhaps ironically, the British National Health Service got out well ahead of U.S. medicine in setting up a P4P scheme for British general practitioners (GPs). The new GP contract listed a series of guideline recommendations that GPs were expected to meet, and specific bonus payments for meeting the goals; and to assure physician buy-in, the government prepared to pay out relatively large sums of money as bonuses in the early years of the contract.

At one level, the experiment worked splendidly. The GPs did such a good job of meeting their goals that the bonuses paid out nearly broke the bank of the health budget; GPs generally earned a bonus of nearly one-third of their previous pay. But that, by itself, ought to send up a red flag. If the very smart people who designed the contract and the P4P reimbursement felt so sure that adherence to the guidelines could only reach a certain level, and the GPs exceeded that level in the first year of the contract, it could mean that the GPs did remarkably well—or it could mean that the GPs figured out a way to game the system. The study provided at least some worrisome suggestions that the latter explanation was correct. The most obvious way to game the system was to use a loophole in the measurements, by which GPs could alter the denominator of their practices. They could, for instance, claim that 10 percent of their diabetic patients had unusual problems with their diabetes, or very difficult life situations, such that it was medically unrealistic to expect them to meet the desired outcome standards for blood sugar control.

In that case these 10 percent of patients would be excluded from that measurement and the bonus would depend on how well the GPs did on the remaining 90 percent of patients. Excluding the maximum number of patients in this way was the best way to guarantee a large bonus. And indeed the study found a direct correlation between the percentage of patients excluded and the amount of bonus paid.[36]

This, of course, is only one attempt to implement P4P, and it occurs in a completely different health-care setting from U.S. practice. What of efforts to implement physician-level P4P reimbursement on this side of the pond? In general, the evidence has not been reassuring. Most experiments to date are very small in scale, quite unlike the British GP contract. They have, as a rule, produced minimal if any changes in practice, compared to the cost.[37] Some P4P plans were found to pay out relatively large sums to reward the already-highest-performing physicians for doing just a little bit better, while the lowest-performing physicians did not improve at all.[38]

We should note what appears to be an inherent problem in any P4P system that takes the general form of the British GP contract. In order to allow precise measurements of outcomes, arbitrary targets are set. For example, the physician may be rewarded based on the percent of patients with hypertension who, after drug therapy, maintain a systolic blood pressure of 140 or lower. Imagine now two hypertensive patients. One is already taking one medicine for blood pressure, and has achieved a systolic pressure of 145. The second has not been given any medicine, and now has a systolic pressure of 180. With one or two medications, this person could relatively easily be brought down to 145; but due to the severity of the underlying condition, it would be very hard to reach a pressure below 140.

The P4P system gives the physician a very strong incentive to add a second medicine to the regimen of the first patient, to get the pressure down, say, to 138. How much real benefit to the patient's health accrues as a result? Hardly any, or maybe none at all. Adding a second medicine increases significantly both the costs and the risks of adverse effects. The change in risk of cardiovascular disease at 138 as opposed to 145 is, by contrast, very small.

By comparison, the physician could make a much more marked improvement in the second patient's risk status, yet the physician has exactly zero incentive to invest time and effort to do so. So far as the P4P reward system is concerned, it makes no difference at all if that patient's pressure is 180 or 145. Both are failures; neither reaches the magic cutoff of 140.[39] The fact that such perverse incentives as these *are readily predictable well in advance* of implementation of any P4P system, and yet do not seem to have slowed advocates' enthusiasm for P4P, ought to give us pause.[40]

Why P4P, at the present state of the art, is a bad idea, is nicely summarized by Andrew Auerbach, Seth Landefeld, and Kaveh Shojania. Auebach and colleagues say little explicitly about P4P, and focus much more on measures for reducing medical error; but it seems reasonable to include P4P among the "novel quality and safety strategies" that they discuss.[41] Their basic complaint is the one we began this chapter with—that the too-rapid employment of any of these methods to improve medical quality and safety, without adequate evidence of their own safety and efficacy in the real world, violates the tenets of EBM. Of overly hasty efforts to reduce medical error, they state, "Medical error may be the eighth leading cause of death in the United States, but by proceeding largely on the basis of urgency rather than evidence, we exempt the eighth cause from standards applied to the top seven."[42]

Auerbach and colleagues review a number of specious arguments used to defend a damn-the-torpedoes-full-speed-ahead approach to improving medical safety and quality, including the one just mentioned—that we cannot afford to wait because people are dying. (An analogous argument made for P4P goes, "Why should we go on paying the same for poor-quality care as we do for high-quality care?") A common thread runs through their rebuttals to these arguments. Medical care systems and organizations are vexingly complex. When we intervene in an attempt to improve quality, we fondly imagine surgical precision: that people will act exactly as the planners hope, leaving all other functions intact and unaltered. In the real world of medical care, by contrast, unanticipated consequences and collateral damage are the order of the day. This complexity in turn means that opportunity costs often dictate whether or not an intervention makes sense. It is not simply the case that we need evidence that P4P works as it is intended; we also ideally desire evidence that P4P improves quality more than any alternative use of the substantial money and energy needed to implement it.

Auerbach and colleagues note that one argument used to short-circuit the difficulties and expense of getting really good evidence before implementing a quality-improvement scheme is that we can do just as well through the emulation of a handful of successful organizations ("best practices"). They note the fallacy of assuming that the factors that actually make the organization successful are indeed the factors that we seek to make others emulate. It is very easy to confuse the cart with the horse. The institution might have tried a P4P experiment and demonstrated improved quality of care, but the P4P success might have been the result, and not the cause, of the improvement in quality.

For an example of this problem, we can return to the case of the British GP contracts.[43] Before the NHS could implement this complicated P4P scheme, it was essential that all British primary-care practices be computerized—an advance that, as of today, has occurred in only a small percentage of American primary-care offices. We do not know how much of the improved adherence to practice guidelines occurred because of P4P, and how much because of the computerization of patient records. If we had to guess, it would seem that the computerization and similar preliminary practice-organization reforms explain the lion's share of the improvement. This may be why the actual improvement in guideline adherence was much greater than the NHS had budgeted for, and the cost of paying the promised bonuses in the first year of P4P put the NHS into red ink.[44]

## :: P4P and Professionalism

A different reason why we should be quite skeptical about P4P proposals has not, to my knowledge, been voiced explicitly, but should be of special interest to bioethics.

Physicians, and especially medical educators, have paid considerable attention to "professionalism" during the last decade. There are various ways this term can be defined.[45] One common element in most definitions is a distinction between a professional role and a purely business role. The professional, it is said, has a fiduciary duty to further the interests of the patient (or client, more generally), which is supposed to predominate over any impulse to maximize profit. It is by contrast quite permissible for a business relationship to be dominated by each party's legitimate desire to make the maximum profit, as long as one avoids outright fraud and other unethical or illegal practices. The term "fiduciary" implies that the professional–client relationship should be one based on trust and trustworthiness; this is quite different from the rule of *caveat emptor* that supposedly governs a business relationship.[46]

At first glance, this would seem to establish a considerable gulf between a professional conception of the physician's work and the basic concept underlying P4P. The physician-as-professional is supposed to do what is best for the patient. She is not supposed to ask if she will be paid more or less for doing what's best for the patient; her professional obligation is to do it regardless. The basic assumption underlying P4P is that physicians respond to financial incentives and, for all practical purposes, only to financial incentives. If you want better care, you will have to pay extra for it; if you do not pay extra, do not expect the physician to adhere to the desired guidelines. In short, at this basic level, there is complete opposition between the concept of professionalism and the presuppositions underlying P4P.

Once we have pointed out these very basic conflicts between the two conceptual schemata, we are hardly done with the matter. It is all very well to say that physicians aspire to be professionals and not *mere* businesspeople. Unless we concoct a system whereby all physicians have other sources of income and pursue medicine as a hobby, it is unavoidable that in some sense, we must regard medical practice as a business. Since medicine is a business at least to some degree, then we should expect that by adopting good business practices, physicians could do their work better, benefitting both them and their patients. We have, for instance, raised the possibility that some of the benefits attributed to P4P in the United Kingdom might rather have been due to early and widespread adoption of electronic health records. Electronic records might benefit physicians and their office staff by making their work much more efficient and less burdensome, and may benefit patients by improving the quality of care. Arguably, the move toward the electronic health record comes primarily from the world of business; it is an attempt to apply to medicine a model of information technology that has proven helpful in many other industries. The electronic record is not a panacea, and there are ways to mess up by using these records. But overall I approve strongly of their adoption, and this would seem to commit me to the position that some business-style reforms can aid medicine.

Once we note first that some business methods may improve medical care for both physician and patient, we might next note that some financial incentives that influence doctors today seem notably perverse and ought to be eliminated. The overly cozy relationship between the pharmaceutical industry and the medical profession is only one case in point. Doctors who do the bidding of the industry, prescribing the greatest quantities of the most expensive drugs, can be rewarded in quite a variety of ways, and in fact considerably magnify their income. In 2007, it was reported that the top orthopedic surgeon on the list of those receiving payments (alleged to be kickbacks for using a certain company's medical devices exclusively) received $1.9 million, while the best-paid child psychiatrist who served on Minnesota's Medicaid formulary committee received $350,000 in speakers' and consulting fees from the drug companies that manufactured the medicines that the formulary committee was supposed to regulate.[47] It seems self-evident to many that if we want physicians to serve the interests of patients rather than the profits of industry, we ought to begin by eliminating these perverse incentives. But once we have made such an argument, can we draw some logical bright line between eliminating perverse incentives and creating virtuous incentives? Have we not, in effect, brought P4P in through the back door?

I have no final answer to offer. On one hand, I am worried that adopting P4P as the savior for assuring quality in the future amounts to undermining the very notion of medical professionalism. On the other hand, I am aware that the arguments I employ might not hold up logically if worked out completely to their conclusions. All I need to show here, however, is that this is a debate of substance, a debate worth having. At present I see no signs of anyone engaging in this debate. And I am aware of no contributions that bioethics is making to identifying the debate as one worth pursuing.

## :: Conclusion

Based on this admittedly brief survey, I conclude that EBM and P4P are significant ethical issues in medicine today. EBM is quite promising in many ways, but is often poorly understood—and the skills of logical analysis that bioethicists bring to the table are precisely the skills needed to better understand and make good use of EBM's potential. P4P, on the other hand, if implemented as rapidly as many today call for, stands to do a great deal of harm—at least as much harm as most worrisome new medical technologies that bioethicists commonly obsess over. How, then, are we to explain the general lack of interest in these topics in our field?

In Chapter 1, I introduced the compelling metaphor suggested by Hilde Lindemann—that medicine is gendered masculine and bioethics is gendered feminine.[48] As feminine pursuits get little respect in our culture, bioethics tries to do its best to act masculine. What we now need to add to the analysis is that medicine is not homogeneous. Different specialties within medicine are gendered differently.

If masculinity is equated with "hard" science, precise quantitative methods, and frequent use of machines and procedures, then subspecialties like surgery and invasive cardiology represent the masculine side of medicine. Society shows that it agrees with this assessment by granting more power and prestige to these specialties, and assuring that their incomes are proportionately higher. By contrast, primary care seems to be the side of medicine most concerned about talking with and listening to patients and forging long-term relationships with patients. This, in the common parlance, is obviously "women's work." It gets much less respect, and the primary-care fields are reimbursed much less well as a result.[49]

If bioethics is worried about its own status, it will want to consort as much as possible with the "masculine" side of medicine, and not be seen in the company of the "feminine" side. This dictates that bioethics will generally ignore primary-care issues. As I assess bioethics over the past two decades, this hypothetical model seems to describe exactly what has happened.[50]

In this and in the previous chapter, I have argued that extremely important ethical concerns are located in areas of medicine that predominantly affect, and that are currently being actively addressed by, the primary-care specialties. These concerns demand both theoretical sophistication—what do we mean by the *best* evidence?—and ultimately highly practical solutions—what specific payment incentives for physicians lie on either side of the line separating professional from unprofessional behavior? As long as bioethics devalues these parts of medicine, the field will remain oblivious to some of the most pressing and intriguing ethical matters.

NOTES TO CHAPTER 4

1. To mention one example, a relatively preliminary and tentative "ethics manifesto" on P4P, from the American College of Physicians ethics committee, appeared only in December, 2007, after most of the writing of this chapter had been completed; Snyder L, Neubauer RL. Pay-for-performance principles that promote patient-centered care: an ethics manifesto. *Ann Intern Med* 147:792–4, 2007.
2. See, for example, Guyatt G, Rennie D, eds. *User's guide to the medical literature: a manual for evidence-based clinical practice.* Chicago: AMA Press, 2002.
3. There is an interesting analogy between this second feature of EBM and the way that the ethical system of casuistry was practiced in its medieval heyday. Albert Jonsen and Stephen Toulmin noted that the classical

casuists appended to each case judgment an explicit assessment of the level of confidence they felt in that judgment: Jonsen AR, Toulmin S. *The abuse of casuistry*. Berkeley, CA: University of California Press, 1988. The analogy is of interest especially since one thoughtful critic of EBM, Mark Tonelli, suggests that EBM ought to adopt a casuistic method for integrating disparate warrants for clinical actions; Tonelli MR. Integrating evidence into clinical practice: an alternative to evidence-based approaches. *J Eval Clin Pract* 12:248–56, 2006.

4. Brody H, Miller FG, Bogdan-Lovis E. Evidence-based medicine: watching out for its friends. *Perspect Biol Med* 48:570–84, 2005.

5. For an example of a history of EBM that appears to appreciate the academic power struggle involved, see Daly J. *Evidence-based medicine and the search for a science of clinical care*. Berkeley, CA: University of California Press, 2005. For a social science study that addresses EBM as if the power in question were spread uniformly throughout medicine, instead of being held by specific medical subgroups, see Mykhalovskiy E, Weir L. The problem of evidence-based medicine: directions for social science. *Soc Sci Med* 59:1059–69, 2004.

6. Thomas L. The technology of medicine. *N Engl J Med* 285:1366–8, 1971. This essay was later reprinted in Thomas's widely read volume, *The lives of a cell: notes of a biology-watcher*. New York: Bantam Books, 1975:35–42.

7. An excellent history of medicine's response to polio in the mid-twentieth century is Oshinsky DM. *Polio: an American story*. New York: Oxford University Press, 2006.

8. The Cardiac Arrhythmia Suppression Trial (CAST) investigators. Preliminary report: effect of encainide and flecainide on mortality in a randomized trial of arrhythmia suppression after myocardial infarction. *N Engl J Med* 321:406–12, 1989.

9. Freedman B. Equipoise and the ethics of clinical research. *N Engl J Med* 317:141–5, 1987.

10. Brody H, Miller FG, Bogdan-Lovis E. Evidence-based medicine: watching out for its friends. *Perspect Biol Med* 48:570–84, 2005.

11. Flexner A. *Medical education in the United States and Canada*. New York: Carnegie Foundation, 1910. The twentieth century was "post-Flexnerian" only in a distorted sense, as few of the so-called Flexnerians ever showed any signs of having read the Flexner report. For example, the dominant mode of medical instruction during most of this era was forcing students to memorize large quantities of scientific facts, a method that Flexner opposed.

12. Engel GL. The need for a new medical model: a challenge for biomedicine. *Science* 196:129–36, 1977.

13. Montgomery K. *How doctors think: clinical judgment and the practice of medicine*. New York: Oxford University Press, 2006. It is of some interest that one of the most sophisticated philosophical accounts of medical epistemology and uncertainty has come from the pen of a literary scholar.

14. Montgomery K. *How doctors think: clinical judgment and the practice of medicine*, pp. 88–9. Montgomery in turn cites Wisdom J. *Paradox and certainty*. Oxford: Blackwell, 1965, p. 138.

15. "[W]here EBM continues to be preached, its continuing attraction appears to remain based on some clinicians' need for certainty in the inherently uncertain world of clinical practice"; Miles A, Polychronis A, Grey JE. The evidence-based health care debate—2006. Where are we now? [editorial introduction and commentary]. *J Eval Clin Pract* 12:239–47, 2006.

16. To give just one example of this, a group of EBM experts, proposing a standardized framework for grading quality of evidence, note a number of concerns about RCTs, and admit that in some circumstances and for some clinical problems, well-designed observational studies may be superior to RCTs. They then proceed to summarize their recommendations in a box that states unequivocally that a randomized trial is "high" on the evidence scale and an observational study is "low." GRADE Working Group. Grading quality of evidence and strength of recommendations. *BMJ* 328:1490, 2004.

17. One example of this argument is: Kassirer JP. Managing care—should we adopt a new ethic? *N Engl J Med* 339:397–8, 1998.

18. Those who believe that bioethics itself needs to focus more on human populations and less on individuals might not be at all bothered by this charge against EBM; see, for instance, Wikler D. Presidential address: bioethics and social responsibility. *Bioethics* 11:185–92, 1997; and Francis LP, Battin MP, Jacobson JA, et al. How infectious diseases got left out—and what this omission might have meant for bioethics. *Bioethics* 19:307–22, 2005.

19. Brody H, Miller FG, Bogdan-Lovis E. Evidence-based medicine: watching out for its friends. *Perspect Biol Med* 48:570–84, 2005.

20. "[I]t seems extraordinary that so much argument continues to take place, that so many medical education curricula continue to change with reference to EBM criteria and that so much clinical practice has been altered—all on the basis of a concept underpinned by an absolute lack of evidentiary basis"; Miles A, Polychronis A, Grey JE. The evidence-based health care debate—2006. Where are we now? [editorial introduction and commentary]. *J Eval Clin Pract* 12:239–47, 2006.

21. Grossman J, MacKenzie FJ. The randomized controlled trial: gold standard, or merely standard? *Perspect Biol Med* 48:517–34, 2005.

22. It is here that "personalized medicine," discussed in Chapter 3 as an imitator of patient-centered care, is said to offer promise. Eventually we will discover the specific gene sequence that causes this individual to respond differently from his fellows, perform the right genetic test beforehand, and therefore know for certain how to treat him. That of course assumes that genetic factors explain all such idiosyncrasies, and that the needed genetic testing is both technically feasible and affordable.

23. Guyatt G, Rennie D, eds. *User's guide to the medical literature: a manual for evidence-based clinical practice.* Chicago: AMA Press, 2002.

24. Tonelli MR. Integrating evidence into clinical practice: an alternative to evidence-based approaches. *J Eval Clin Pract* 12:248–56, 2006. As noted previously, Tonelli believes that a variant on the casuistic method from ethics would best serve EBM in this regard.

25. Goldenberg MJ. On evidence and evidence-based medicine: lessons from the philosophy of science. *Soc Sci Med* 62:2621–32, 2006, quote on p. 2622.

26. Goldenberg MJ. On evidence and evidence-based medicine: lessons from the philosophy of science, quote on p. 2624, citation omitted.

27. Goldenberg MJ. On evidence and evidence-based medicine: lessons from the philosophy of science, quote pp. 2630–31, italics in original.

28. Brody H. *Hooked: ethics, the medical profession, and the pharmaceutical industry.* Lanham, MD: Rowman and Littlefield, 2007, esp. pp. 97–116.

29. Lexchin J, Bero LA, Djulbegovic B, Clark O. Pharmaceutical industry sponsorship and research outcome and quality: systematic review. *BMJ* 326:1167–70, 2003.

30. Tyson J. Evidence-based ethics and the care of premature infants. *Future Child* 5:197–213, 1995; Tyson JE, Stoll BJ. Evidence-based ethics and the care and outcome of extremely premature infants. *Clin Perinatol* 30:363–87, 2003.

31. Loughlin M. A platitude too far: "Evidence-based ethics." Commentary on Borry (2006), evidence-based medicine and its role in ethical decision-making, in *Journal of Evaluation in Clinical Practice* 12, 306–311. *J Eval Clin Pract* 12:312–18, 2006.

32. Borry P, Schotsman P, Dierickx K. Evidence-based medicine and its role in ethical decision-making. *J Eval Clin Pract* 12:306–11, 2006.

33. Loughlin M. A platitude too far: 'Evidence-based ethics,' pp. 312–8.

34. Loughlin M. A platitude too far: 'Evidence-based ethics,' quote on p. 316.

35. For an example of enthusiastic endorsement of P4P based on this study, see Epstein AM. Paying for performance in the United States and abroad [editorial]. *N Engl J Med* 355:406–8, 2006.

36. Doran T, Fullwood C, Gravelle H, et al. Pay-for-performance programs in family practice in the United Kingdom. *N Engl J Med* 355:375–84, 2006.

37. One study of P4P applied at the hospital level looked at the differences in mortality outcomes between hospitals that stood at the 25th and the 75th percentiles for compliance with several widely used evidence-based guidelines, for treatment of pneumonia, heart attack, and heart failure. The authors found that there was indeed a statistically significant difference between the high- and low-performing hospitals; but that the differences amounted to about one percentage point, and were for all practical purposes negligible. If one were to base Medicare P4P on these measures, as many have actively encouraged, the actual payoff in terms of patient outcomes would be minuscule compared to the costs of implementing such a major change in reimbursement. Werner RM, Bradlow ET. Relationship between Medicare's hospital compare performance measures and mortality rates. *JAMA* 296:2694–2702, 2006.

38. Rosenthal MB, Frank RG, Li Z, et al. Early experience with pay-for-performance: from concept to practice. *JAMA* 294:1788–93, 2005; Glickman SW, Ou FS, DeLong ER, et al. Pay for performance, quality of care, and outcomes in acute myocardial infarction. *JAMA* 297:2373–80, 2007.

39. I am grateful to Jerome R. Hoffman for emphasizing this risk of P4P guideline targets.

40. One might object that all that is needed here is a bit of fine-tuning of the targets. One could pay a certain bonus amount for the patients who achieve a target at or below 140; and a second bonus amount for all the remaining patients who achieve a pressure below 150, for example. But this "solution" is really only more of the same. The problem still is that continuous variables that determine health risks and health outcomes are ignored so that we can focus on arbitrarily chosen dichotomous variables. The problem is not solved, merely relocated.

41. Auerbach AD, Landefeld CS, Shojania KG. The tension between needing to improve care and knowing how to do it. *N Engl J Med* 357:608–13, 2007, quote on p. 608.

42. Auerbach AD, Landefeld CS, Shojania KG. The tension between needing to improve care and knowing how to do it, quote on p. 608 (citation omitted).

43. Doran T, Fullwood C, Gravelle H, et al. Pay-for-performance programs in family practice in the United Kingdom. *N Engl J Med* 355:375–84, 2006.

44. Auerbach et al. also observe that once an institution has tried a new quality-improvement measure, such as P4P, and has had short-term success, it has two options. It can aggressively promote itself based on this purported success; or it can be scientifically skeptical and rigorously measure its outcomes to see whether the success is real and how long it lasts. The average organization has every incentive to do the former and few to do the latter; Auerbach AD, Landefeld CS, Shojania KG. The tension between needing to improve care and knowing how to do it, pp. 608–13.

45. When I began work on this manuscript, I had intended to include a chapter specifically on professionalism, partly because of the challenges for ethical analysis posed by uncertainties and ambiguities in definition. This chapter was, eventually, excluded from the present volume, due mainly to difficulties in having it cohere sufficiently with the remaining chapters. If pressed, however, I would certainly include professionalism in the agenda for "the future of bioethics," as I believe that it requires in many ways a fresh look and fresh methods. See also Chapter 12.

46. Medical professionalism project. Medical professionalism in the new millennium: a physicians' charter. *Lancet* 359:520–2, 2002; Rhodes R, Cohen D, Friedman E, et al. Professionalism in medical education. *Am J Bioeth* 4(2):20–22, 2004; Stern DT (ed.) *Measuring medical professionalism.* New York: Oxford University Press; 2006; Cohen JJ. Viewpoint: linking professionalism to humanism: what it means, why it matters. *Acad Med* 82:1029–32, 2007.

47. Bollier J. Investigators: Dr. Jeffrey McLaughlin received more than $600,000 in payments. *Oshkosh* [WI] *Northwestern*, December 2, 2007; Associated Press. Financial ties link docs, drug companies: Minn. Law shines light into money big pharma spends on panel members. MSNBC.com, August 21, 2007, http://www.msnbc.msn.com/id/20379563/(accessed January 2, 2008).

48. Lindemann H. Bioethics' gender. *Am J Bioeth* 6(2):W15–W19, 2006.

49. On the widening gap between incomes in primary care and other specialties, see Bodenheimer T, Berenson RA, Rudolph P. The primary care-specialty income gap: why it matters. Ann Intern Med 146:301–6, 2007. Indeed the disparity is becoming so severe that Bodenheimer and others predict a crisis, as medical students actively avoid primary care career slots and a severe shortage of primary-care physicians looms.

50. At the risk of stretching the metaphor farther that it should go, I note that the one book that I am aware of, that purports to address EBM from an ethical and philosophical standpoint, is actually more about computers in medicine than about EBM—as if the only legitimate way to discuss EBM in bioethics is through a discussion of machines; Goodman KW. *Ethics and evidence-based medicine: fallibility and responsibility in clinical science.* New York: Cambridge University Press, 2003.

# 5 ::

# Community Dialogue

Mr. Smith lies in the intensive care unit. There is a dispute about whether he should be maintained on a ventilator, or started on renal dialysis. Would these measures be of benefit to him? Would they merely prolong the dying process? We bioethicists are called to the bedside for a consultation.

Our initial response to the consultation request will be both unanimous and vociferous. Let Mr. Smith speak for himself. We must hear the voice of the patient—the voice that for too many decades or centuries, the paternalistic practice of medicine sought to ignore or suppress. As the playwright eloquently phrased it: Whose life is it, anyway?[1]

Perhaps we will find upon further inquiry that the voice of Mr. Smith cannot now be heard. Perhaps he is comatose or delirious. In that event, ironically, we demand even more that we somehow manage to find his voice and listen to it. Perhaps he has executed an advance directive. Perhaps he had conversations about his wishes with his loved ones. Perhaps twenty years ago he once made a passing comment to a stranger on the street. No matter; we will move mountains to find that voice and then to listen to what it said.

I caricature here, of course. But I also, for the most part, approve.

But now, let Mr. Smith arise from his bed. Let him put on his clothes and walk out of the hospital. Let him go about his daily business in the community. Suddenly, our bioethicists' insistence that his voice be heard dissipates. In our bioethics work, we read what each other has written; we teach our classes using each other's textbooks; we attend conferences to listen to each other speak on panels; we form committees among ourselves; and we tell the world the right answers. Nowhere in the process does the voice of Mr. Smith seem to play a role in how we conduct our business.

Let Mr. Smith do one more thing. Let him stand outside the nursing home where Terri Schiavo lies, in what the experts call a persistent vegetative state, and what her parents insist represents a slow but inexorable recovery. Let Mr. Smith wave a picket sign, and declaim loudly to the television crews that experts like us are murdering Ms. Schiavo. At this point our bioethicists' interest in hearing Mr. Smith's voice reaches an all-time low.[2]

We bioethicists have not always and everywhere behaved like this. At one point, there were so many of us running about the country, trying hard to locate Mr. Smith and to listen to his views, that we spoke of "the grassroots bioethics movement."[3] The grassroots effort was largely focused on one ethical question—access to health care. This focus made good sense, theoretically, in a democratic society with an overriding individualist culture. It made sense to ask Mr. Smith, and no one else, what kind of medical care he should receive; and it made sense to ask the mass of Mr. Smiths what all of them thought about what policy their government should follow in securing access to health care. A conservative critic of bioethics would, I imagine, reply, "There goes bioethics being liberally biased again." Everyone knows that liberals support the right to decide on life-prolonging treatment, especially if one decides to refuse it; and everyone knows that liberals support a role for government in health care. To the conservative, it sounds as if bioethics likes to hear Mr. Smith's voice only as long as he agrees with us.

Today, we seldom hear anyone mention any "grassroots" movement. Yet here and there, interesting work is being done that shows that our ability to elicit Mr. Smith's voice on bioethical matters has actually gained sophistication since the 1980s. This chapter is a review of some of those developments, and a plea to return the "grass roots" to a more central role in our theoretical and practical work.


## ∷ Grassroots Bioethics

Bruce Jennings, surveying the grassroots scene for the *Hastings Center Report* in 1988, dated the inauguration of the movement four years previously: "In the spring of 1984, news was moving eastward about an innovative program under way in Oregon known as Oregon Health

Decisions. By organizing participatory forums at the grassroots level throughout the state, the Oregon project seemed to bridge the gap between health care provider and consumer groups, and between experts and 'ordinary' citizens."[4]

Between 1985 and 1987, the Prudential Foundation devoted a quarter of a million dollars to Community Health Decisions, supporting efforts like Oregon's in California, Hawaii, Idaho, Iowa/Illinois, Maine, and Washington.[5] The Robert Wood Johnson Foundation funded the ongoing efforts in Oregon as well as new programs in New Jersey and Vermont.

Jennings summarized the experience:

> The mission of community health decisions projects is to stimulate a well-informed conversation where many voices are heard and all reasonable perspectives are given due consideration. It is important to note that the projects remain neutral on the controversial topics they bring before the public through community forums and other activities. Some may be skeptical about the possibility of achieving this kind of fairness and neutrality. The Community Health Decisions movement is proving the skeptics wrong. These projects are demonstrating that it is possible to provide forums for citizen education and dialogue without imposing hidden agendas on the participants, and without trying to manipulate the outcome of the process.[6]

He went on to describe a key achievement, and also to distinguish the community dialogue concept from more usual social science research methods:

> One of the most noteworthy achievements of these projects is their ability to create forums where differing points of view can be heard in an atmosphere of constructive dialogue and mutual respect. Careful records of these deliberations have been maintained by project staff. In most cases, questionnaires have been used to gauge participants' opinions and preferences. Such surveys cannot claim rigorous scientific validity. But unlike most polls, they tend to reflect opinions that have been informed and shaped by participation in a prolonged and serious discussion of the issues. These results may indicate more reflective and deliberative views than those growing out of broader, randomly selected, but less participatory opinion surveys.[7]

The *Hastings Center Report* next addressed the grassroots bioethics movement in 1990. Michael Garland, bioethicist and then-president of Oregon Health Decisions, described what his organization had done following the passage of a 1989 law providing for the Oregon Medicaid health-rationing plan. The law required that the state prioritize medical treatments, with the understanding that the lowest-priority treatments would not be covered under the Medicaid system for the state's poor. Oregon Health Decisions convened 47 meetings around the state to inquire of citizens what moral values should guide this prioritization scheme. Garland described the resulting value choices, but also admitted the worrisome facts that 93 percent of the attendees at the meetings were Caucasians, and 70 percent were college-educated.[8] It did not appear that it was necessarily the Medicaid enrollees themselves who were helping to decide what treatments ought or ought not be provided through Medicaid.

Garland suggested in this brief article that the special accomplishments of Oregon Health Decisions would be the eventual determination of an ethically sound and politically acceptable prioritization scheme for the state's Medicaid program. He did not say (but could have) that the value of Oregon Health Decisions had already been demonstrated by the fact that the legislature passed the law in 1989. Oregon became the only state to pass what we might argue was a *uniquely bioethically informed* piece of legislation. Today the "R word," rationing, is still viewed as a deadly third rail by any politician daring even to contemplate health care reform. Yet, nearly 20 years ago, the politicians in the Oregon legislature accepted a law that stated openly, first, that rationing would be necessary if all lower-income people in the state were to have access to basic, decent health care, and second, that the state's leaders had to bite the bullet and create an *explicit, public* system of rationing for which they could then be held accountable.

It seems quite unlikely that such a bill could have passed the legislature without the work of Oregon Health Decisions in organizing community dialogues, culminating in a statewide health-care constitutional convention. Somehow the Oregon voting public had been convinced that the politician's standard stump speech on health care, promising many things, blaming the standard villains, and tackling none of the really hard choices, was poppycock. Somehow the politicians must have gotten the message that if they did not talk sense and grapple with the real problems, they were going to lose votes. The creation of this pool of shrewd, well-informed voters was perhaps Oregon Health Decisions' greatest achievement.[9] This achievement stands despite the later sad fate of the Oregon Medicaid system.[10]

By January, 1993, when the newly elected Bill Clinton set out to tackle serious national health care reform, there was therefore an existing model of how one might approach health policy through the vehicle of community dialogue. Clinton himself liked the town meeting format and, to many observers, especially displayed his talents in that sort of forum. Unfortunately, when Bill and Hillary Rodham Clinton set out to create the process to launch health reform, they looked too far northward on the Pacific coast. Instead of looking for inspiration to Oregon Health Decisions, they picked as their health reform guru Ira Magaziner, who had worked with such businesses as Boeing. Magaziner implemented an expert-driven model that helped condemn the Clinton Health Plan even before it could gain traction, by giving the impression that it was the creation of a secret elitist cabal.

The ultimate failure of the Clinton health plan in 1994 might have led to the conclusion that the Clintons had the right basic idea, but used the wrong means to move it forward—and would have done much better had they relied on a grassroots approach. Instead, the conclusion many drew was that comprehensive health reform is simply a political nonstarter. Whether as a result, or for other reasons, one heard little of "grassroots bioethics" after that.

## ⠶ Theoretical Concerns about Consensus

One general response that the field of bioethics has had to public bioethics of all sorts—including both community dialogue and grassroots efforts, as well as governmental bioethics commissions—is to ask what moral authority or warrant such deliberations carry.[11] Jennings, for example, describes competing models of consensus and discusses the conditions that must be met for consensus of the right type to have a "justificatory role in ethics."[12]

For our purposes in this chapter, I propose to cut the Gordian knot and suggest that these theoretical questions are largely beside the point. I am willing to grant, for purposes of discussion, that the fact that a particular viewpoint on a bioethics question emerges from a process of community dialogue grants that viewpoint no moral warrant or authority whatsoever. Instead, that viewpoint gains moral traction exclusively on its own merits. Discussions of consensus often assume the value of some form of ethical shortcut—that once one knows that a position is a consensus position, something else follows without a need for further justification. For community dialogue to yield the benefits that I will argue for, no such shortcut need be contemplated. Community dialogue is quite capable of yielding the wrong answer to a bioethical question, and any community dialogue process is quite capable of correction and refinement to an indefinite degree. The extent to which the results of a community dialogue carry moral weight is something that cannot be determined prior to observing and questioning both the result and the process that led to it.[13]

## :: Models for the Community Dialogue Process

While leaving the problem of consensus aside, it is nevertheless worth considering some models that have been proposed for the conditions and methods that will lead to the best outcomes for community dialogue. What sort of bioethics practice is required to make this endeavor succeed?

A point of departure is the model we might call "democratic consensus," developed by Jennings and informed by the first round of grassroots bioethics activities in the 1980s.[14] Jennings identified the following characteristics of the process:

- We agree that we lack an independent source of moral truth, since appeal to that source would obviate the need for any
  further dialogue.
- A special space is created for participation and dialogue.
- The dialogue experience occurs within the larger context created by democratic institutions and practices. (For instance, dialogue participants need not fear that when they leave the dialogue space, they might be subjected to physical reprisals for participating or for expressing certain opinions.)
- The participants are viewed as free and equal within the process.
- The participants engage seriously in the dialogue—that is, they are open to the possibility that their moral identities and values may be transformed as a result of the exchange.
- The dialogue is restricted to the giving of reasons; considerations labeled as "irrational" are excluded.

The outcome of the process is viewed as a set of policy recommendations. The dialogue participants are not seen as themselves writing or developing policy; rather they produce a set of prioritized moral values of a sort useful for directing and informing policy. (In any event, the outcomes are supposed to be practically useful; the participants do not see themselves as merely entertaining each other with abstract speculations.)

As a next iteration, Leonard Fleck summarized his own experience with Community Health Decisions–type projects in 1992.[15] Fleck initially described his model as "informed democratic consensus," later employing terms such as "informed democratic deliberation" or "rational democratic deliberation."[16] Fleck accepted all the criteria suggested by Jennings with the following added features:

- The dialogue is informed by accurate scientific information.
- The dialogue is guided by facilitators trained specifically in ethical discourse.
- Participants are broadly representative of the community.
- Participants view the outcome of dialogue as an explicit, binding choice. They are willing to live with the consequences of the values and priorities they advocate, as those consequences would affect their and their loved ones' future lives. (That is, they approach the dialogue process with the appropriate degree of moral seriousness.)

More recently, Catherine Myser has proposed a model for community dialogue that is drawn from a different intellectual source—the social-science model of community-based participatory research.[17] A purported strength of this model is that it is aimed specifically at increasing diversity, by facilitating input from minority communities that might otherwise be overlooked or excluded. The community-based participatory research model adds some features to the models we have previously reviewed, but also disagrees with some features required by those other models. The new features proposed by community-based participatory research include:

- Professional "experts" and members of the community collaborate in defining the questions to be addressed by the dialogue.
- The products of the dialogue are disseminated for the use and benefit of all parties (for example, they are not taken away to be published by the "experts" in an academic journal that will be read only by other academics).

These new features are aimed at assuring that the dialogue process is *democratic* in a deeper sense. They point out ways in which, however well the "experts" design a process by which all participants are treated as free and equal *within the dialogue space,* as soon as the parties leave that space, inequalities of education and status may take over and create circumstances in which the community participants may feel that they have been used or exploited by those who convened the process. The community-based participatory research model is in that regard a more rigorously egalitarian and anti-elitist model.

The community-based participatory research model rejects one condition called for by the previous models: "The dialogue is restricted to the giving of reasons; considerations labeled as 'irrational' are excluded." However well-intentioned, such a condition may create a non-level playing field in a community whose members have been brought up in ways different from the majority community. They may not have had the formal education that gives one facility and fluency in expressing complex judgments in sequential, logical form. They may also have had much more experience in settings where wisdom is imparted by means of narrative, drama, song, ritual, and other means of communication that the majority community labels as "emotional" and therefore, "irrational." The advocate of community-based participatory research argues that we can have all the benefits sought after by the reasons-only clause, without its downside, if we altered the condition to the following: "The dialogue is open to all *mutually respectful* forms of expression."

Community-based participatory research also departs from the previous models in one other way. True to its origins as a social-science research tool, the model refuses to adopt as a condition that "participants view the outcome of dialogue as an explicit, binding choice."

The final model I will consider is *community-based dialogue.*[18] This model grows out of a dialogue project that involved communities of color in discussions of genetic screening and the related issues of genetic privacy. As it involved minority communities, the level-playing-field advantages claimed for the community-based participatory research were clearly attractive. Yet the advocates for this final model agreed with Jennings and Fleck that it was essential that the dialogue process be an *ethical* exercise, and not some sort of participant-observer research. For that reason, the community-based dialogue model reinstates the requirement that community-based participatory research had rejected—that participants view the outcome of dialogue as an explicit, binding choice.

Table 5.1 summarizes all four models.[19]

TABLE 5.1 Comparisons Among Community-Dialogue Models

| | Democratic consensus | Informed democratic consensus; rational democratic deliberation | Community-based participatory research | Community-based dialogue |
|---|---|---|---|---|
| Lacks an independent source of moral truth | X | X | X | X |
| Special space is created for participation | X | X | X | X |
| Occurs within democratic context | X | X | X | X |
| Participants viewed as free and equal | X | X | X | X |
| Participants engage seriously | X | X | X | X |
| Dialogue restricted to giving of reasons | X | X | | |
| Outcome: policy recommendations | X | X | X | X |
| Informed by accurate science | | X | X | X |
| Guided by trained facilitators | | X | X | X |
| Participants broadly representative | | X | X | X |
| Participants bound by outcome | | X | | X |
| Experts, community collaborate on defining questions | | | X | X |
| Products disseminated for good of all | | | X | X |
| Open to all mutually respectful expression | | | X | X |

## ⁑ Outcomes of Community Dialogue

While these models are no doubt interesting, the question obviously arises—what, exactly, is the practical outcome of the process that makes this extensive effort appear to be worthwhile? The outcomes would, of course, be of little value or interest if one could predict them. Typically, when community dialogue in bioethics has been conducted previously, extensive records of the deliberations were generated. To give a complete account of the outcomes of any such dialogue process would go well beyond the space allowed in this chapter. On the other hand, a quick summary of the dialogue results would tempt the skeptical reader to say, "So what is so wonderful about that? I could have thought all those things up on my own."

By way of illustration, consider the outcomes of the Communities of Color and Genetics Policy Project, conducted jointly by the University of Michigan, the Michigan State University Center for Ethics and Humanities in the Life Sciences, and the Tuskegee University National Center for Bioethics in Research and Health Care (2001).[20] This three-year project, funded by the Ethical, Legal, Social Implications of the Human Genome Project (ELSI, NIH), engaged fifteen dialogue groups, each consisting of fifteen to twenty participants, in various communities in Michigan and Alabama. The sites were selected to include both African-American and Hispanic communities, including members representing lower socioeconomic and educational status.

The project directors took home two major lessons—first, that dialogue works in these settings, that rational discussion of controversial and complex health policy matters can occur despite cultural, educational, and language barriers; and second, that consulting communities of color yielded conclusions that would not necessarily have arisen had the dialogues been conducted only in the majority community.[21]

One key area of discussion was "trust/distrust." The groups concluded that they could not rely solely on either government or private industry to conduct genetic research and testing in the interests of their communities, and recommended that an independent "advocacy group" be created as a watchdog apparatus. Another related area was "education." Perhaps contrasting the intensive front-loading of user-friendly information on genetics that they received as part of this project with their previous level of knowledge, groups argued that it was critical that public education do a much better job in the future of conveying information on genetic technologies and research and the related policy questions.

Concerns about "privacy" of genetic screening results focused on three contexts—privacy within families and among family members; privacy from testing by employers or insurers; and privacy of genetic information within the physician–patient relationship. Discussion of "genetic testing" yielded four major conclusions:

- All genetic testing must be voluntary
- Privacy of genetic test results must be protected
- Access to testing should be assured to all who could significantly benefit
- Access to education and counseling is essential if individuals are to make informed choices about the use of genetic testing

An example of the fineness of grain attainable in these discussions is hinted at by the following summary conclusion: "Germline genetic engineering should be an option available to individuals, but there should be some socially determined limits with respect to how that technology is used. There should be no social policies or practices that endorse the use of germline genetic engineering for eugenic purposes."[22]

The particular report from which these examples are drawn is written to stress specific policy recommendations. Alternatively, one could have structured the report to highlight the moral values that underlay the policy recommendations. The designers of this particular dialogue exercise envisioned their task as creating a practical instance of John Rawls's theoretical concept of reflective equilibrium. Rather than reason from specific cases to general moral principles, or vice versa, the participants were provided with an array of concrete cases as well as background information, and encouraged to work both ways. By deciding what moral values seemed to them of highest priority, they might determine what policy to recommend. Alternatively, perhaps only after seeing what practical policy they favored, might they have been able to reason backward to see how they were prioritizing their moral values.[23]

## ⠶ Advantages

The community dialogue experiments conducted so far seem promising enough to suggest that bioethics ought to dedicate itself to the more regular utilization of this method. Beyond the enlightenment that is generated on any specific topic, the following general outcomes are likely.

*Keeping bioethics humble.* Many years of working in the field of family medicine taught me a number of things. Patients in the hospital, lying flat in bed, having to look up to see the physician, and wearing a gown open in the back, may appear to be relatively passive and easily cowed by medical authority. These same patients, wearing their street clothes, walking in under their own power, sitting and staring back at me at the same level, and with places to go and appointments to keep as soon as the office visit is over, can be quite another matter. Those latter patients seldom failed to let me know when they disagreed with me or when they thought my advice inadequate or irrelevant. They often made it quite clear if they had come seeking a specific goal and I had not given them what they wanted. If physicians of any specialty are inclined to arrogance or pomposity, I would suggest a term of duty in family medicine as an antidote.

Bioethics practitioners are not immune to the failing of becoming too full of ourselves. A regular dose of community dialogue for bioethicists might fulfill a similar function as a regular dose of ambulatory primary care for physicians.[24]

*Keeping bioethics connected.* Under the community-based dialogue model, the community representatives and the "experts" collaborate in determining what questions the process ought to address. If (as has usually been the case previously) any given community group engages in dialogue just once, on a preselected topic such as genetic policy or access to health care, there will be little opportunity to make informed recommendations on future discussion topics. If, as I would recommend, community dialogue groups engage in *regular and repeated* dialogues on a *series* of topics or issues, then these groups will eventually become quite savvy about what questions are *not* being asked among bioethicists—even though those questions may be of great concern to the community. The result might drive bioethics in a more engaged, responsive direction.

*Improved public understanding.* I argued above that one notable result of Oregon Health Decisions—even if one not clearly foreseen by its originators—was perhaps the most informed state-wide electorate in the nation on the topic of health care access. If the community dialogue model were replicated widely enough across the country by various bioethics centers, a similar outcome would be an expanded and deeper public understanding of what bioethics is all about. The average person would no longer have to rely upon sensational novels or films to depict the "typical" bioethicist.[25] One might hope eventually for a public that is much better prepared to address bioethical issues that come up in the course of their lives, and who are much less easily stampeded by scare tactics when bioethics-related legislation is being considered.

*Novel insights.* Bringing a different set of voices to the table, and conducting discourse in a way quite different from standard academic discussions, ought over time to yield genuinely new ways of seeing important bioethical issues. As community participants gain in sophistication, they will also suggest for discussion ethical questions that had simply never occurred to us to *be* bioethical issues. Paul Farmer and Nicole Gastineau Campos suggest that bioethics would be quite a different enterprise if we had a way of routinely tapping into the views and critiques of the sick poor of the developing world, to whom most of today's bioethical deliberations seem both irrelevant and silly.[26]

*Novel hypotheses.* Important new hypotheses will be generated if dialogue on the same issue is conducted simultaneously by a number of different community groups, and the groups reach quite different conclusions. What factors led to this diversity of opinion—racial, ethnic, or cultural differences, socioeconomic or educational differences, differences in the dialogue process at various sites, or chance alone? Further, systematic exploration of these potential explanations might shed important light on the issue.

## ⠔ The Problem of Representativeness

When the idea of community dialogue is raised with an audience, one of the first questions almost always asked is how the organizers can be sure that the participants in the dialogue are truly representative of the community in question. Obviously, two methods that we employ to assure representation of the community in other contexts—a community-wide election, and random, scientific sampling—are not available for this purpose.

Previous grassroots bioethics exercises made no special effort to assure that groups were representative. Rather, a high level of interest in the process, and a willingness to engage in the procedures that had been agreed upon, took priority. In some cases, such a focus on active participation rather than representativeness backfired, as when the groups in Oregon that helped determine what the Medicaid rationing system would look like included very few individuals who would be eligible for Medicaid.

To some extent, we can defuse the issue of representativeness by refusing to claim any special moral warrant for the group's conclusions. Nonetheless, a more rather than a less representative set of participants from the community is obviously desirable if the objectives of dialogue are to be achieved. Several methods can be used. A community advisory board can be convened to help plan the dialogue sessions, and that board charged explicitly with trying to enhance the representativeness of the proceedings. The dialogue process can be publicized by local newspapers and radio stations, with clear instructions on how to be included. Meetings can be open to all willing onlookers, even those who do not wish to actually engage in the process (for example, by reading the materials provided before each session).

I suspect, in practice, that representativeness will be an iterative process and a moving target. The first several dialogue sessions held in any particular community might draw those most active and interested. If the results are adequately publicized within the community, complaints will be voiced through various channels if any segment of the community sees itself as having been excluded. Such objections will then lead to invitations to join further dialogues, and perhaps to modifications such as changing the venue or the timing of the sessions to allow those previously excluded to attend. There seems to be more to be gained by starting the process of dialogue at the community level, and committing ourselves to continuous improvement in the representativeness of the participants, rather than refusing to even begin the dialogue until we have evolved a foolproof plan to assure representativeness.

There are several reasons why the home visit has almost completely died out in American medical practice. There is the technological reason that we imagine that you cannot provide adequate medical care without a lot of "stuff." That stuff lives in the physician's office, and it is logistically difficult to lug it around while visiting the patient's home. Then there is the financial reason that the travel time in going to and from home visits is simply not reimbursed at a rate anywhere near what that same physician's time could generate if she were in the office seeing more patients. Despite all these reasons, experienced primary-care physicians know that you can learn things about the patient by visiting him just once in his home environment, which you could never learn in a dozen office or hospital visits.

Bioethicists need not replicate the old-fashioned physician's house call. But we should, I suggest, make it more of a regular practice to seek out Mr. Smith and his neighbors when he is not hospitalized, and see what they have to say about a number of subjects. We would find that we can learn things that way that we would never find out in dozens of hospital consultations.

NOTES TO CHAPTER 5

1. Clark B. *Whose life is it anyway?* New York: Dodd, Mead, 1979.
2. For the disputes related to the case of Ms. Schiavo, see, for instance, Schneider CE. Hard cases and the politics of righteousness. *Hastings Cent Rep* 35(3):24–7, 2005; and other commentaries in the same issue.
3. Jennings B. A grassroots movement in bioethics. *Hastings Cent Rep* 18 (3, suppl) 1–15, 1988.
4. Jennings B. A grassroots movement in bioethics, quote on p. 1.
5. According to project snapshots provided by Jennings, most of these programs in states other than Oregon were confined to a region of one or several counties, and were not statewide; Jennings B. A grassroots movement in bioethics.
6. Jennings B. A grassroots movement in bioethics, quote on p. 5.
7. Jennings B. A grassroots movement in bioethics, quote on p. 6.
8. Garland MJ, Hasnain R. Health care in common: setting priorities in Oregon. *Hastings Cent Rep* 20(5):16–8, 1990.
9. As an individual case study, consider John Kitzhaber. Before Oregon Health Decisions, he was a little-known emergency room physician. As a result of his participation in the program, he became a leader of the Oregon senate, and later governor, and a nationally recognized authority on health policy.
10. On the eventual failures of the Oregon Medicaid rationing experiment, see Oberlander J. Health reform interrupted: the unraveling of the Oregon Health Plan. *Health Aff* 26(1):w96–w105, 2006.
11. Moreno JD. *Deciding together: bioethics and moral consensus.* New York: Oxford University Press, 1995.
12. Jennings B. Possibilities of consensus: toward a democratic moral discourse. *J Med Philos* 16:447–63, 1991. Jennings considers a pluralistic consensus model and an overlapping consensus model and argues instead for consensus as it emerges from "dialogic democratic practice."
13. The discussion here could be expanded and refined. One of the most interesting outcomes of community dialogue, of the sort to be described

below, occurs when we succeed in bringing to the table voices that are not usually heard from, and the resulting conclusions reflect the input from those voices. That is, we can see, in hindsight, that we would not have reached those conclusions had a certain process of inclusivity not been followed. In this situation, it is too facile to say that the conclusions possess moral weight only on their own merits. Rather, there is a reciprocal relationship between the process and the outcome; each reflexively lends additional credence to the other. This happy outcome cannot, however, usually be determined or predicted in advance.

14. Jennings B. Possibilities of consensus: toward a democratic moral discourse.
15. Fleck LM. Just health care rationing: a democratic decision-making approach. *U Penn Law Rev* 140:1597–1636, 1992.
16. Fleck LM. Just caring: Oregon, health care rationing, and informed democratic deliberation. *J Med Philos* 19:367–88, 1994; Bonham VL, Citrin T, Warshauer-Baker E, et al. *Community based dialogue: engaging communities of color in the U.S. genetics privacy conversation* (in press); Fleck LM. Creating public conversation about behavioral genetics. In: Parens E, Chapman AR, Press N, eds. *Wrestling with behavioral genetics: science, ethics, and public conversation*. Baltimore: The Johns Hopkins Press, 2006, pp. 257–85.
17. Myser C. Community-based participatory research in United States bioethics: steps toward more democratic theory and policy. *Am J Bioeth* 4: 67–68 2004.
18. Bonham VL, Citrin T, Warshauer-Baker E, et al. *Community based dialogue: engaging communities of color in the U.S. genetics privacy conversation* (in press)
19. References for each model are cited in the text above. Not all of the elements marked with an "X" in Table 5.1 are explicitly mentioned by each author. For the sake of simplicity, I have indicated that an element is part of the model if it seems consistent with the spirit of the model and is not explicitly rejected by the author.
20. The complete materials may be found at http://www.sph.umich.edu/ genpolicy/current/reports/index.html (accessed March 18, 2007).
21. http://www.sph.umich.edu/genpolicy/current/reports/index.html (accessed March 18, 2007).
22. http://www.sph.umich.edu/genpolicy/current/reports/summary_ dialogue_report.pdf (accessed March 18, 2007); quote on p. 6.
23. Fleck LM. Creating public conversation about behavioral genetics. In: Parens E, Chapman AR, Press N, eds. *Wrestling with behavioral genetics: science, ethics, and public conversation*. Baltimore: The Johns Hopkins Press, 2006, pp. 257–85.
24. Community dialogue, conducted regularly, could help protect bioethics from Carl Elliott's fear of the arrogance that accompanies being placed in a bureaucratic role with the presumption of expertise: Elliott C. The tyranny of expertise. In: Eckenwiler LA, Cohn FG, eds. *The ethics of bioethics: mapping the moral landscape*. Baltimore: Johns Hopkins University Press, 2007, pp. 43–6.

25. For a fascinating account of several sensationalist portrayals of bioethicists in popular novels, see Klugman CM. The bioethicist: superhero or supervillain? *ASBH Exchange* 10(1):1, 6–7, 2007.
26. Farmer P. Campos NG. New malaise: bioethics and human rights in the global era. *J Law Med Ethics* 32:243–51, 2004.

# 6 ::

## Overview: Bioethics, Power, and Learning to See

This chapter lays out a conceptual model that will be used in the next four chapters. The model is derived from one form of feminist ethics and addresses an aspect of power disparities that, if not understood, could undermine careful ethical reflection. I will then proceed to apply some aspects of this model to cross-cultural issues, race and health disparities, disabilities, and international health justice.

### :: Moral Development and "Learning to See"

Judy Andre argues that an important part of moral growth and development is "learning to see."[1] A good deal of bioethics is written as if the central problem were reasoning correctly from given facts to the desired moral conclusions. That model presumes that the facts are indeed given at the outset—that is, all discussants are aware of the facts and would readily agree on what they are. When we are spoon-fed "the facts" in a typical bioethics textbook case presentation ("The patient is a 67-year-old woman who completed an advance directive ten years previously..."), the notion is reinforced that "the facts of the case" are there for the asking.

Andre counters that a good deal of unethical behavior arises, not from poor reasoning, but rather from a perceptual problem, a moral blindness. We simply *do not see* that the case in front of us is this sort of case; or that we stand in such-and-such a relationship to the person with whom we interact. Making moral progress in our lives, learning to behave better where previously we behaved poorly, is as much a matter of fine-tuning our moral perceptions, "learning to see," as it is of honing our reasoning skills.

Sometimes, learning to see simply requires new experiences and new insights. We may never have thought of certain possibilities before. The value of literature in teaching ethics is precisely this opportunity to introduce us, in a compelling way, to many more life experiences and varieties of human relationships that we could ever experience at first-hand in a single life-time. "In a compelling way," here, means that literature has the power to force certain perceptions on us, when other modes of presentation might allow us to erect psychological barriers. Some perceptions are painful. Fearing pain, we often avoid going down a pathway that would lead us to novel ways of perceiving the world. Good literature breaks down these defenses, and forces the perception on us before we anticipate which way the path is headed and before we can put up our shields.[2]

In other instances, learning to see is harder. There are times when we (usually unconsciously) *choose* not to see. At these times, we have a strong reason for wishing to see the world in a certain way and in not wanting to allow a divergent perspective to enter our conscious-ness. This is especially true when we are comfortable with a pattern of behavior, and when perceiving the world differently would cause us to seriously question the correctness of that entire pattern of long-standing, habitual behavior. In such a case, the act of seeing, finally, is life-changing. One can never go back to the prior state of ignorant bliss. One may decide, in the end, to keep on acting in the same old way and to follow the same old patterns. But now one is forced to admit that one has made a *conscious* choice to do so. One has to accept moral responsi-bility for that conscious choice. It was much easier in the old days, when the comfortable pattern of behavior seemed perfectly natural and when no other way of behaving had suggested itself.

An example of this phenomenon might be a person who has been in the habit of telling racist jokes. Very likely the behavior was learned from his elders, and for a while, no one on his social circle seemed in any way offended or upset by these jokes. So he has no conscious awareness of any moral issues raised by telling these jokes. Eventually, a friend becomes irate and expresses offense when he tells one of these jokes. The joke-teller has now come to a fork in the road. He could elect no longer to tell such jokes in the future, which is tantamount to admit-ting that he has been unwittingly engaging in racist behavior for his entire previous life. Or he could elect to continue to tell such jokes. In either case, he has to own responsibility for making an explicit choice. It is highly tempting to try to find a way to deny that this moment of realization has arrived—such as to blame the friend and to claim that it is simply her problem, as she obviously has no sense of humor.

## ∷ Feminist Insights Regarding Power

Feminist ethics has been extremely helpful in teaching us to see through one particular type of moral blind spot.[3] This moral blind spot is typified by gender relationships in a traditional male-dominated society. It could, however, be described more generally as a set of social arrangements characterized by a social power hierarchy, in which two groups occupy one-up and one-down positions in relation to each other.

One variant of feminism teaches us that the world looks very different depending on whether one is a member of the (relatively) powerful or the powerless group. The more powerful group sees the world as an orderly place in which each group of people occupies the place assigned to it by natural laws. Those who have more power and authority in this society are motivated primarily by reason and kindness, and exercise their power for the overall good of society—including the best interests of the less-powerful group. When histories of the society are written, they focus on the doings of the people in the more powerful group, since they were the ones making the important decisions and guiding the destiny of the society. Members of the less-powerful group performed very important tasks, of course, but their role was secondary and supportive.

The "cult of domesticity" that describes social patterns in the Victorian era is a typical case study of this way of seeing the world. The public life of Victorian society was a man's world. Women were excluded from this world not by prejudice or discrimination, but by nature. They were hampered by conditions such as childbirth and menstruation, and were naturally emotional rather than rational creatures, unsuited for the worlds of business, government, and academia. History books told of wars and battles, heroes and leaders who were almost always male. Women belonged in the private sphere of hearth and home, where their peculiar skills and talents could be used to the best effect—rearing children, and influencing their husbands gently to soften some of the less desirable, masculine rough edges while providing loving support and refuge from the pressures of the world. Women should be content to occupy that realm; seeking a more public role for themselves was a sign of psychopathology.

The world appears a very different place to the group that occupies the one-down power status. This group notes that many of the actions of the dominant group seem anything but kind, generous, and public-spirited. Members of this group know that many of them are quite capable of occupying roles in society that are traditionally allocated to the more powerful. The rules that exclude them from these roles appear arbitrary and unjust, not a working-out of the natural order of the universe. Members of this group know all the ways in which the society would grind to a halt if they were to cease their contributions—their work in child-rearing, for example, or even something as simple as mopping the floors and doing the laundry. Yet they never see those tasks talked about in the public life of the society with the respect or credit due them. So far as the literature, or the history, or the laws of the society would tell the story, these tasks, and the people who do them, simply are invisible.

When members of the one-down group attempt to confront the more powerful group with their perceptions, they encounter a dismissal that takes the form of bemused puzzlement. Their narratives of their lives and experiences, and of their future aspirations, are treated as what Hilde Lindemann Nelson calls "damaged" narratives.[4] It is simply taken for granted by their listeners that what they are saying cannot be right or true, and that the tellers of these narratives are perceiving the world in a basically incorrect fashion. When they say, for instance, that women could become business executives or world-class athletes, it is just as if they were saying that the earth is flat and the moon is made out of green cheese. The only people who would tell such damaged narratives must be mentally and morally inferior. That inferiority is taken by the more powerful group as further evidence why power can never be safely entrusted to the one-down group, and why the more powerful group must continue to exercise power on behalf of their weaker and less capable compatriots.

If I, as a member of the more powerful group, can be encouraged to see the world in the way that the one-down group sees it, then important changes in perspective occur. Ways of behaving that previously seemed enjoyable and innocent may now appear to me to have serious consequences for others' well-being. Things that I did in the past, for which I assumed that I was owed full credit because of my individual efforts, may now be seen as having arisen at least in part from my special position of privilege in the society, and I have to admit that equally talented and hard-working members of the one-down group were denied the same opportunities that I took as my due.

To me as a member of the more powerful group, achieving this new perspective is a profoundly disturbing experience. In some ways, I am now forced to revise my autobiography. I can no longer see myself as quite the same person I thought I was. It is no wonder that I might resist mightily the moment of insight that would force these unpleasant and burdensome conclusions on me.

Again employing an example from race relations, a typical way for me to respond to my own life circumstances is to give myself full credit for being admitted to and then graduating from college. I studied diligently in grade school and passed the standardized admission tests with good scores. It is hard to get me to imagine what the world would have been like for me had all the following been true:

- My own parents had never attended college and so could offer no advice or assistance with practical tasks such as college applications.
- My social peer group treated college attendance as deviant and suspect behavior.
- I attended inferior public schools that did a very poor job of preparing me for college.
- The standardized tests had been designed for a "normal" group of students who were culturally and perhaps linguistically different from me.
- The college admissions process contained numerous, unconscious discriminatory features, such as favoring children of alumni of the college, and in the past, those attending the college had almost always been from a different racial group.
- No one in my or my parents' social circle had any connections with the college, so no one could be asked to intercede personally on my behalf.

If I could be helped to see the world as it would be seen by an 18-year-old with all those attributes, then perhaps I might get my first glimpse of what the concept of "white privilege" means.[5] The revelation could be profoundly painful, as I would then have to confront how much of the success that I had uncritically ascribed to my own accomplishments was actually due to forces over which I had no control. Small wonder that some bioethicists, when confronted with a possible role for "whiteness studies" in their field, respond by deriding the very notion.[6]

## ⋕ Autonomy: Bioethics' Solution?

The feminist model of how the world looks different to those on opposite sides of social power disparities ought to be especially appealing to bioethicists. The modern phase of bioethics, starting roughly in the 1960s and 1970s, dealt with precisely that sort of power disparity. Insight in that world of bioethics involved "learning to see" past the blinders that that power disparity had placed upon the eyes of physicians.

Physicians and patients, according to an oversimplified version of bioethics' genesis narrative, occupied positions somewhat analogous to men and women in Victorian times. Physicians took it for granted that they were justified in exercising power over their patients based on their medical knowledge, their experience and wisdom, and their benign motives. Patients, if left to their own devices, were far too ignorant and fearful to make prudent decisions about medical treatment. It was much better for the patients that physicians should choose for them in a paternalistic mode—indeed, that was what the vast majority of patients explicitly wished for. (The very word "paternalism," which bioethics adopted to characterize this newly discredited physician–patient relationship is rather self-consciously adapted from the role of *paterfamilias* in the traditional Victorian social world.) And the final consequences of this paternalistic system of medicine were happy patients and generally correct therapeutic decisions.

The bioethics movement of that day—made up of both outsiders to medicine, first theologians and later philosophers, plus a few forward-looking, rebellious physicians—proved successful at ripping the blinders off medicine's comfortable, one-up power position. Physicians were forced to *see* that other, darker motives were at work alongside their benevolence; and that the consequences of paternalistic decision-making were often undue suffering, especially at the end of life when newer medical technologies were overused or misapplied. In a nutshell, the "new" bioethics was extremely successful.

The intellectual sword that the bioethical St. George used to slay the dragon of medical paternalism was the principle of respect for autonomy. In a Kantian move, bioethics turned the tables on the paternalistic physician by focusing attention on the basic commonalities of the respective positions of physician and patient. Paternalism depended on seeing primarily the differences between the patient and the physician—the patient scared and ignorant; the physician placid, knowledgeable, and experienced. Respect for autonomy required rewriting this narrative so that both patient and physician emerged as potential rational decision-makers, each with certain definite but non-overlapping areas of expertise and information. The physician might be an expert in what side effects a drug might cause and how frequently they occur; only the patient is an expert on what the occurrence of such a side effect might mean for his or her life. (Mark Siegler educated his fellow physicians on this point by elaborating a case of a ballet dancer with asthma. The steroid medications that best controlled her asthma caused muscle weakness that interfered with the finer movements required at her level of dance artistry. She eventually decided that she would rather be a superb dancer who wheezed, than someone who could breathe without difficulty but who could not dance well.)[7]

This overly compressed description of the early days of bioethics suggests both why the autonomy "movement" won out, and why so much of later bioethics has been devoted to undoing some of the collateral damage. Physicians and patients are similar in important ways, and they are different in important ways. A comprehensive ethics of medicine takes both similarities and differences fully into account. A limited, Kantian focus on the principle of patient autonomy is therefore far from a comprehensive medical ethic.

But for our purposes in this chapter, the more important lesson that bioethics took away from the "paternalism wars" of its early days was that *the principle of autonomy resolves problems of power imbalance*. In hindsight, we now see that this picture was seriously incomplete. What made it seem a relatively easy victory, that both physician and patient could be viewed as rational decision-makers occupying roughly equal positions of power, were the unspoken background assumptions that both physician and patient were:

- male (or sufficiently male-like so that gender did not matter)
- white
- English-speaking
- temporarily able-bodied

In a roughly analogous fashion, it was easy to argue the principle of "one man, one vote" in the early days of the American republic, as long as everyone understood that the vote would never be extended to blacks, women, American Indians, and other "inferior" groups.

With the comfortable assumption that invoking the principle of respect for autonomy automatically creates a level playing field, bioethics was saved for years from having to confront the tough question: *when does the very act of invoking autonomy privilege the status of white, English-speaking, temporarily-able-bodied males; and systematically disadvantage others?*

The first group of scholars within bioethics to ask this tough question were the feminists. Feminism, with regard to autonomy, has gone both ways. At one level, feminist criticism of the dominant medical practices was content to invoke the principle of autonomy, and merely to insist upon its wider application. For example, calling attention to the moral personhood and rights of the pregnant woman is in many ways a sufficient reply to a medical view of reproductive decision-making that reduces the pregnant female to a system of organs with the uterus in the center.[8]

Another sort of feminist criticism cuts deeper, at least for the purposes of this chapter. An example of this deeper criticism is Margaret Urban Walker's *Moral Understandings.*[9] If we survey the entire fabric of human life, and list all of its ethical features, we see that a narrow swath of it consists of relative strangers encountering each other, and having to appeal rationally to rules and principles to resolve conflicts and disagreements. Within that narrow swath of human life, appeals to the principle of autonomy work just fine. But outside that narrow world of what Walker calls the "theoretical-juridical model" of ethics, is all of the rest of life—what, the wag says, happens to us while we are busy making other plans. Walker reminds us that a very large swath of life consists of important human relationships, in which the pertinent moral tasks are, not to reason from rules and principles, but rather to understand each other and to treat each other responsibly. In this much wider arena of life, appeals to the principle of respect for autonomy do much less useful work. By contrast, narrative tools that examine the sorts of stories we tell about others and about ourselves, and how we reason from those stories to what ought best to happen next, have much wider applicability.

Rita Charon tells the following story from her medical practice. An architect, a long-time patient, had received embolization treatment for a cerebral hemangioma, but unfortunately the mass had regrown. The patient asked for an appointment to discuss two surgical options, each with serious risks.

Relationship

[S]he reported in great detail the opinions of her neurologist and neurosurgeon. She described the results of magnetic resonance angiography (MRA) scans and the like, but I didn't want to see the studies or read the reports. I did not feel the need to perform a physical examination, nor even to check her blood pressure. Instead, we sat together, close to one another, as she told in detail what she was going through and I listened...I wanted to let her *hear* herself tell of what the judgments were, what they meant, which of the several scary things she feared the most. I wondered myself how angry she felt that this thing she thought she had bested had come back.

As we sat in my office, I understood that she wanted both my internist's brain and my narratologist's brain. I understood the pact we had made that, by my hearing her out, she would hear herself out.... We appreciated the time-bomb nature of this reoccurrence, the singular details of her own work situation, and how the possible operative complications would interfere with her work, and attempted to look full in the face all the uncertainties incumbent on any course of action, including doing nothing. We relied on our own inter-subjective history as patient and doctor, realizing that our previous truth-telling and mutual confirmation were now, when she needed it, paying off. Because she felt free to say *fully* what was in her to say, I could take the measure of her fear, her courage, her resilience, her lack of blame, and her tremendously brave awareness of the possibility for grave losses. I, meanwhile, fulfilled my ethical duties toward my new knowledge of her situation by offering to contact a renowned hematologist at another institution whose research might contribute to the patient's decision-making. As we left my office, we both bowed our heads to signify that we had done important, serious, and moving work together, all of it narrative, all of it medical, all of it mutually constitutive of ourselves.[10]

The theoretical-juridical model is very clear on what this encounter is "about." It is all about informed consent, or shared decision-making, or perhaps in the older locution, patient education. (As a primary-care physician, the way that I would document the visit in the chart, to justify billing for the time I had spent, would be, "Spent 60 minutes with the patient, more than half of which was counseling and/or coordination of care.") Dr. Charon obviously respected the patient's autonomy fully, so ethically there is little to be said about the case.

Ethically, there is a great deal to be said about this "case," and Charon leaves much of it unsaid in the end. What was the almost-holy presence before which she and the patient instinctively bowed their heads? What exactly had happened during this period of time, and how was each of them changed as a result of it? They certainly did not, as the visit concluded, worship at the altar of informed consent. (We must nevertheless remember that, had other physicians *not* respected the patient's right of informed consent, this extremely important and valuable encounter would never have happened.)

The standard conceptual tools that we associate with informed consent and respect for patient autonomy cannot do *full* justice to this encounter. Walker would say that this is because Dr. Charon and her patient approach each other as friends rather than as strangers. To explain exactly what *sort of* friends they are—I would imagine, for instance, that they probably have no social contacts outside of the medical practice—would require a good deal of elaboration. But the basic point is that they aspire to some level of intimacy. A relationship ethic rather than a stranger ethic is needed to describe what sort of encounter this is. To adopt William May's resonant phrase, Dr. Charon is trying to find the best way to "rise to the occasion."[11] That is a different matter from seeking to do her duty or to respect the patient's rights. Without a richer or a more extended narrative, perhaps one written jointly by the physician and the patient, we will not be able to plumb this ethical question to the bottom.

## ⠏ Bioethics' Future Agenda

My argument so far may be summarized:

1. Bioethics ought to be concerned with power disparities within society, and the impact that these disparities have on individuals involved in health-care relationships.
2. Bioethics over the past three decades has relied especially on one tool to address power disparities—appeals to the principle of respect for autonomy.
3. Feminist bioethicists have shown us in a compelling way that gender inequalities persist and are not resolved merely by appeal to autonomy, however useful autonomy can be within the appropriate ethical sphere. In the process, feminists have reminded us of how much of human ethical life exists outside of the sphere of rules and principles.
4. We now need to apply those same bioethical insights to power disparities that arise due to cultural and racial/ethnic differences, and that are experienced by persons with disabilities and by citizens of developing countries.
5. Having addressed those other power disparities, we also need to return to health care itself, to see whether "autonomy" has actually

been as successful in empowering the patient as it was supposed to be. (My answer, as explained in Chapter 3 when we addressed patient-centered care, was "no.")

This chapter has been predominantly a theoretical exercise, extending a conceptual tool initially developed for gender relationships in society to deal with other types of social relationships. As we address the specific topics in the next several chapters, we will need to ask the twin questions: What further *theoretical* refinements are needed for bioethics to address that set of issues satisfactorily? How will the *practice* of bioethics change if the field embraces that set of issues?

NOTES TO CHAPTER 6

1. Andre J. Learning to see: moral growth during medical training. *J Med Ethics* 18(3):148–52, 1992.
2. One way to view this dynamic, suggested by the work of Wayne Booth among others, is that when we read fiction, we form a relationship with the author/narrator. We decide that we can trust this individual sufficiently to travel for a while in her company and to allow her to show us the world as she interprets it. That level of presumed trust in the narrator may be responsible for our willingness to open ourselves to novel interpretations and perceptions. Booth WC. *The company we keep: an ethics of fiction.* Berkeley: University of California Press; 1988.
3. I am grateful to Susan Squier for the reminder of the many variants of feminism that I am excluding from consideration here, in order to focus on a single concept derived from feminist work that seems to me to be most applicable to the issues that I want to address. While I make no claim to expertise in feminist studies, it would seem that the model that I present here regarding power disparities between social groups is an element of, or derived from an element of, feminist standpoint theory. At any rate, standpoint theory is categorized as a feminist epistemology, and the use that I wish to make of this model is primarily epistemological— that we will know the world in a very incomplete way if we listen only to the more powerful of the social groups. The model does not address any of the various feminist issues that follow from standpoint theory, or that would probably be classified as part of postmodern feminism. On these matters generally, see Kemp S, Squires J. Section 2: Epistemologies: introduction. In: Kemp S, Squires J (eds.) *Feminisms (Oxford readers).* New York: Oxford University Press, 1997, pp. 142–5. It may be of interest to note an important analogy between bioethics as I here describe it, and Kemp and Squires's account of feminism—that it is by its nature both interdisciplinary and emancipatory in its goals.
4. Nelson HL. *Damaged identities, narrative repair.* Ithaca, NY: Cornell University Press; 2001.

5. Jensen R. *The heart of whiteness: confronting race, racism, and white privilege.* San Francisco: City Lights; 2005.

6. Navel-gazing: bioethics and the unbearable whiteness of being [editorial]. *New Atlantis* (2):98–100, 2003. This was a response to Myser C. Differences from somewhere: the normativity of whiteness in bioethics in the United States. *Am J Bioeth* 3(2):1–11, 2003. For other reactions, see the extensive comments published in the same journal issue.

7. Siegler M. Searching for moral certainty in medicine: a proposal for a new model of the doctor–patient encounter. *Bull NY Acad Med* 57:56–69, 1981.

8. I have heard it reported that one widely used mid-twentieth-century obstetrical textbook referred to the pregnant female as "the gravid uterus and its support structures." I have been unable to locate this precise wording. Hahn noted that early editions of *Williams Obstetrics* referred to a woman in terms such as "the maternal organism" and "the generative tract"; Hahn RA. Division of labor: obstetrician, woman, and society in *Williams Obstetrics*, 1903–1985. *Med Anthropol Q* 1 (new series):256–82, 1987. I am very grateful to Julie M. Trumble, Moody Medical Library, University of Texas Medical Branch, for research assistance on this question.

9. Walker MU. *Moral understandings: a feminist study in ethics.* New York: Routledge; 1998.

10. Charon R. *Narrative medicine: honoring the stories of illness.* New York: Oxford University Press, 2006, p. 59.

11. Quoted in Frank AW. *The wounded storyteller: body, illness, and ethics.* Chicago: University of Chicago Press, 1995, p. 62. Frank in turn cites May WF. *The patient's ordeal.* Bloomington, IN: Indiana University Press, 1991, p. 131.

# 7 ⸬
# Cross-Cultural Concerns

Despite the lack of specific index listings in the recent *Oxford Handbook of Bioethics*, more attention is being paid to cross-cultural or multicultural issues in bioethics.[1] To pay attention, those practicing bioethics had to overcome two formidable obstacles. The first was a general distrust of the social sciences and of any of its empirical research as relevant to bioethics. The second was analytic philosophical ethics' dismissal of culture as irrelevant, since any true ethical statement ought to take the form of a universal proposition that holds for all cultures and all historical periods. An increased comfort with interdisciplinary approaches to bioethics that include the social sciences, and the acceptance of alternative ethical approaches that focus on moral particulars rather than universals, were therefore essential first steps.

In this chapter I will offer a few introductory remarks about what "culture" is. I will then take up in turn two theoretical concerns. The first is a move to preserve the ethics-as-universal approach by insisting that universals can accommodate all important aspects of culture. The second is the apparently opposite move to turn ethics entirely over to culture in the name of ethical relativism. Finally I will look at two case studies for cross-cultural bioethics—female genital mutilation or cutting; and international research ethics—to suggest some of the practical applications of these theoretical moves.

## ⠇ Problems in Defining "Culture"

The term "culture" is often flung about quite loosely. I will not devote space here to giving a detailed definition, except to note two observations that help to keep some of the most common misconceptions at bay. First, culture is porous and dynamic. This has been true historically and it is even more true today in an era of ubiquitous electronic information exchange. "Culture" does not equal "fixed, immutable tradition." Second, we are all multicultural beings. Through the course of our lives we live in multiple worlds, usually in several at the same time, each one with a discernible and often distinct culture. For example, an adult actively involved in the spheres of home, church, and workplace might be said to participate in three different cultural worlds. It is crucial to shed the myth that we modern people of the West are somehow acultural as we go about our business, and only encounter culture when we come into contact with someone "exotic" from a distant and more primitive part of the world.[2]

From what vantage point does medicine address cross-cultural issues? Maya Goldenberg offers a perspective from philosophy of science, which suggests that there is something fundamentally dishonest about how medicine deals with culture. Even though many sciences, especially the social sciences, have come to embrace post-modernist views of scientific objectivity and value-freedom to varying degrees, medicine (as noted in previous chapters) seems still wedded to a positivist view of science. On this view, the scientist-physician is a dislocated, disinterested, and ultimately invisible observer who has the capacity to perceive the external world as it really is. The post-modern critic recognizes this person, the autonomous knower, as having ideals of rationality, objectivity, and value-neutrality that are typical of modernism. In turn, these ideals can be shown to be rooted in a view of the world that is uniquely European, professional, and masculine. But those same ideals prevent this invisible knower from seeing himself as situated in such a social context. Instead, according to these ideals, this knower inhabits the "culture of no culture."[3]

If I am going to interact with people from a different culture, it would seem an excellent starting point to be fully aware of my own cultural allegiance and its roots. Medicine provides its inhabitants with a very poor starting point, by contrast, if its very ideology requires that they deny their cultural location and identity. This denial seems to have two levels. First, we deny that medicine itself is a culture and that its practitioners act in certain ways and believe certain things as a result. We therefore forget that someone coming from a different culture (even though that might be the dominant culture within our society) might experience the encounter with medicine as jarring and dislocating. Second, the culture-of-no-culture ideology causes us similarly to think wrongly about our own cultures of origin, before we became members of the medical profession. Whatever I was before I became a physician, the scientific training that I underwent cleansed me of it, leaving me some sort of purified human being. It is therefore from a vantage point of pure scientific rationality that I approach the patient, who is so unfortunate as to be immersed in his own culture. As medical anthropologists like to describe our fallacies, we physicians imagine that only exotic or weird people have "cultures"; normal people do not.

## ⠃⠃ Bioethics: Universal or Pluralistic?

Raanan Gillon has become a champion of a universal, or what he calls "culturally neutral," approach to bioethics, the "four principles plus attention to scope." He begins by adopting Beauchamp and Childress's well-known four principles of bioethics: respect for autonomy, beneficence, non-maleficence, and justice: "The four principles plus scope approach claims that whatever our personal philosophy, politics, religion, moral theory, or life stance, we will find no difficulty in committing ourselves to four *prima facie* moral principles plus a reflective concern about their scope of application. Moreover, these four principles, plus attention to their scope of application, encompass most of the moral issues that arise in health care."[4]

Gillon offers as an example of how "scope" applies to health-care ethics the problem of respecting the autonomy of pediatric patients. Older children are fully capable of autonomous choices that we can readily agree we ought to respect. Very young children lack virtually all capacity for autonomous choice. Children in a middle age range fall somewhere in between and may call for novel approaches. Gillon suggests, "It is salutary to reflect that these contentious issues are not about the content of our moral obligations but about to whom and what we owe them."[5] In what way this is salutary, or why, is not explained.

It is instructive to contrast Gillon's approach with that of Godfrey Tangwa. Tangwa, an African philosopher, is concerned about implications of the philosophical systems of his native continent for the practice of bioethics. He notes that there is no single, unified and cohesive "African philosophy," but contends that there are sufficient similarities among the indigenous philosophical systems of the various African peoples to allow some generalizations.

Tangwa identifies two specifically African threads that would, if understood and adopted, take bioethics off in rather different directions from its present trajectory. The first is the concept of a person. Most traditional African thought systems ascribe many of the moral features that Westerners attribute to the human individual, to larger collectives such as the extended family or clan. The Westerner sees an individual as a morally autonomous agent; the African views an individual as an incomplete moral being, who can achieve moral wholeness only as a member of the larger collective. The second African thread is the relationship between the human and the natural world; to the African, this connection is much tighter than would be recognized by most Western thought systems.[6]

How well does Gillon's approach assist us in dealing with what Tangwa has proposed? We might first note that Gillon, in claiming that any and all limitations or defects in the "four principles" approach can be remedied merely by adding attention to scope, has stacked the deck in his own favor by selecting certain examples. It certainly seems true that some moral disputes in health care are less about the content of a moral principle and more about the class of individuals to whom the principle applies. For that set of disputes, "principles plus scope" may describe the moral landscape in a helpful way. But it seems unlikely that all moral disputes of interest will fit that tidy pattern, and hence be closely analogous to extending autonomy to young children, for example.

As a first step, one might suggest that the rights of self-determination that we have become used to calling "respect for autonomy" properly belong to the clan rather than the individual. If so, the individual vs. clan dispute is another good example of where "scope" will do the job. We are simply altering the class of entities in the world to whom the concept of "autonomy" applies. But this move does not adequately explain what is at stake in *denying* the relevant aspects of moral autonomy to the human individual, in the process of relocating them to the clan. In the typical Western view, the adult individual human with mental capacities is the paradigm case of what we mean by respect for autonomy. Such an entity is part of the "scope" of the principle of autonomy, if any entity at all is. The puzzlement that is generated by suggesting that the individual human may not be fully autonomous therefore seems to lie well outside of what could adequately be addressed by Gillon's "attention to scope."

But let us imagine that Gillon, after much effort, succeeds in extending his account of the four principles plus attention to scope, so that he can claim to have covered the instances that Tangwa has cited. Perhaps he can bring to bear the principles of beneficence and non-maleficence in explaining why the clan has attributed to it a level of autonomy that the individual lacks, and perhaps he can extend his account of justice so that it includes non-human species. We are still left with the question: so what? What would make us think that Gillon's account is superior to, far less as good as, an account that recognized the ethical pluralism among the systems of thought? On the contrary, we would have every reason to suspect that Gillon has been able to force these African concepts into his Western ethical system only by distorting many of their nuances and subtleties. Yet it is precisely those nuances and subtleties we would attend to, if the objective of bioethics were to see if we could *learn something from* African philosophy—instead of seeking an excuse to dismiss African philosophy. (Recall that, at this point, there is as yet no question of declaring that the African philosophical approach is *correct*. We may still, in the end, reject any system that denies that degree of respect for autonomy to the individual human being. Rather, we are at this stage simply trying to be sure that we fully understand what the African system of thought consists of.)

The dangers of misrepresenting or distorting the other systems of philosophical thought, in order to get them to fit a system such as Gillon's, seem obvious. Why, then, would Gillon and his supporters feel an overriding compulsion to rescue a universal and culturally neutral ethics, whatever its cost?[7] It is certainly true that Anglo-American analytical philosophy, for much of the twentieth century, treated universality as a sine qua non of ethics. Yet there are now several lines of criticism of this ethical love affair with the universal. One, articulated well by Richard Rorty, takes its origins from American pragmatism.[8] According to Rorty, whatever the difficulties in constructing and defending an ethics that is thought to be absolute and universal, many have felt driven to that goal because the only alternative was ethical relativism. Moreover, people assumed that ethical relativism meant that there could be no ethical standards whatsoever and no grounds on which to criticize even the most egregious or evil behavior. This either-or account, Rorty claims, is simply nonsense. Between the unacceptable extremes of absolutism and extreme relativism are many other versions of ethical relativism that have few of the flaws attributed to the extreme version. On careful examination, these moderate forms of relativism turn out to be far more sensible ways to think about ethics than the either-or bogeyman would suggest.

The other line of criticism comes from feminism. Walker, for example, would suggest that Gillon's felt need for a universal, culturally neutral ethics arises from his commitment to what she calls the theoretical-juridical model of ethics.[9] According to this model, the only ethics worthy of the name must consist of abstract, general principles and must be applied to specific cases in a manner somewhat analogous to the function of a court of law. If, however, we survey the entirety of the human moral life, we discover that only a relatively small corner of that life truly demands a theoretical-juridical approach. Much of the remainder is bound up in human relationships and how we act responsibly within those relationships. We ought not try to force the ethics of relationships and responsibility into the theoretical-juridical Procrustean bed. Before we tried to shoehorn Tangwa's African ethical observations into the "four principles plus scope," Walker might rather have us ask whether the African ethical system could represent a type of relationship ethics, focusing on human relationships within a large extended family and relationships among humans and the natural world. The latter approach might enhance our understanding in a way that the former would not.

## ⬌ Ethical Relativism: How Serious an Issue?

Richard Rorty's defense of moderate versions of ethical relativism notwithstanding, some might conclude that by rejecting Gillon's offer of a universal system for health care ethics, I have committed myself to a crude version of ethical relativism, according to which each society or each culture gets to decide on its own grounds what practices are moral or immoral, and members of other cultures have no rational grounds on which to challenge any of those conclusions. Others would argue that even though I may not be committed to this crude ethical relativism, I must at least grapple with it and attempt to refute it, else my project of sketching out a "multicultural bioethics" for the future will come to naught.

Both of these conclusions are misleading. I certainly will not adopt a position of cultural relativism. Nor is it necessary to expend much powder and shot defending any other position from the attacks of ethical relativists.

If Loretta Kopelman is correct, we need simply to stand aside and allow ethical relativism to refute itself. Kopelman notes that the statements that express the position of ethical relativism actually take the form of cross-cultural ethical "truths." If it is wrong for culture A to judge culture B, from culture A's standpoint, then it must be similarly wrong for culture C, D, and so forth to do so. But that is precisely the sort of *cross-cultural* ethical statement that cultural relativism, itself, would exclude. Hence cultural relativism cannot proclaim itself without contradicting itself.[10]

This point is a slight modification of a general response to those who claim to adopt an ethical-relativist posture. There is an old chestnut about how the philosophy classroom teacher should respond to a student who stakes out, in class discussion, a frankly relativist position. She should tell the student that because he has expressed this distasteful and inadequate view of ethics in an ethics class, he has therefore failed the course. The student will then (we can confidently predict) object bitterly to the *unfairness* of her action. The teacher will reply that if he were the ethical relativist that he said he was, he would understand that he would have his views of what grade in a course is fair, that she would have her views, and that no one could have any rational grounds for choosing between them. Since he instead appealed to some criteria for fairness, as something both of them could understand and appeal to, he must not be an ethical relativist after all.

The point of this sophomoric exercise is simply that, while many people talk ethical relativism, few actually believe in or practice it. With a little patient inquiry, the same can be found to be true for "cultural" relativism.

There is one other reason not to worry very much about cultural relativism as an issue that must be "settled" in some definitive manner, before we can have an appropriate multicultural bioethics. Martha Nussbaum, in her approach to justice that we will discuss at greater length in Chapter 10, offers a useful distinction between justifications for criticizing a society or nation for injustices against its own people, and justifications for coercive interventions against such a society.[11] One of the motives for cultural relativism is an abhorrence of nations who take advantage of their military or economic power, to coerce less powerful nations to adopt moral practices or systems that the former approve of. Going to war against an authoritarian regime, in order to impose a democratic regime on a nation that has previously shown little evidence of wanting one, might be an example of this form of neocolonialism.

We can, however, share this abhorrence of neocolonialism, while still holding that another society's political and cultural practices are unjust. If the society is engaging in gross violations of human rights, such as occurred in Rwanda and Bosnia, we might have no choice besides military intervention. But there will be many cases of purported rights violations that do not rise (or sink) to that level. In these other cases we will attempt persuasion and education. We need adopt neither extreme position—either that that culture has the prerogative to treat its people however it wishes, simply because it is a distinct "culture" (whatever that may mean); or that because the culture is treating some of its people unjustly, we are both justified in intervening, and obligated to intervene, coercively in that other nation's affairs.

## ∷ Female Genital Mutilation as a Case Study

Female circumcision or genital mutilation would seem to be a very instructive case study in what approach multicultural bioethics ought to take.[12] The practice drives home Nussbaum's distinction from the previous section—most of the developed world condemns it, but no one, to my knowledge, has proposed armed intervention to stamp it out. The practice also poses the multicultural dilemma in its starkest form—to one side of the debate, it counts as a gross and basic violation of the human rights of its victims; to the other side, objections discount the practice's long tradition and cultural importance, and constitute an especially blatant form of ethical imperialism.

The practice is as slippery empirically as it is ethically. Some authors uncritically run down a laundry list of medical complications of genital mutilation; others argue that this is the same as listing all the known side effects of a drug commonly employed in Western medicine, as if all patients who took the drug suffered from all of these effects. We imagine that there is some connection between this practice and Islamic religious beliefs, however lacking the theological rationale might be for any direct tie between Islam and female circumcision; but others note that the practice is unknown in many Muslim nations, and is practiced among many non-Muslim communities. Some view the practice as firmly rooted in and embodying male domination of women; yet case reports exist of mothers secretly taking their daughters to be circumcised against the vocal objections of the father, and of women in a society being the principal defenders of the practice.[13]

Despite these ongoing controversies, a degree of international consensus has emerged on female genital mutilation. It has been condemned by the United Nations and the World Health Organization. Perhaps more to the point, a protocol on the rights of women in Africa was adopted at a conference of heads of state of the African Union in Maputo, Mozambique, in July 2003. The protocol went into force in November, 2005 when the fifteenth country formally ratified it; as of June, 2006, two additional nations had ratified.[14] Such international instruments make it harder to argue that we are imperialistically imposing Western values on the rest of the world when we oppose the practice. Nonetheless, these legal agreements at the government level do not necessarily correlate with the reduction or disappearance of the practice at the local level. While precise figures are difficult to obtain, and now are perhaps impossible as practitioners fear disapproval or legal sanctions, at least some surveys hint that the prevalence of genital mutilation is actually increasing in some areas—and is moving to the West, along with immigrants from those nations where it is most deeply rooted.[15]

Assuming that American bioethicists wish to condemn female genital mutilation, what specific actions would they then recommend? Effective interventions would seem to require, first, an accurate understanding of the social forces that currently encourage the practice. Recommendations become complicated as one lists the various different reasons given in its favor:[16]

- It is a traditional rite of passage that initiates a girl into womanhood, and signifies acceptance by the adult community of women.[17]
- It guarantees the woman's virginity before marriage, and assures faithfulness and sexual temperance after marriage, along with (in some forms) enhancing the male partner's sexual pleasure.[18]
- It renders the woman beautiful, by removing ugly structures that appear to be derivations of the male genitalia and hence not truly feminine.
- It is believed, probably erroneously, to be required as a matter of religious teaching.[19]
- It is believed, erroneously, actually to improve the health of the married couple.

Generally, more than one reason is given in any community where female genital mutilation is practiced; and as one travels from community to community, or from nation to nation, different reasons may be given primacy. That means in turn that no single intervention is likely to be generally successful in opposing the practice. For instance, some success has been achieved in some locales with alternative womanhood initiation ceremonies. This would be expected to be valuable among people who see initiation as the main reason for genital cutting, but hardly likely to succeed among people most concerned with standards of feminine beauty.

Esthetic justifications for female genital mutilation especially raise problems for American bioethics. American medicine, for supposedly cosmetic reasons, feels fully justified in carrying out potentially painful surgical procedures on the genitalia of non-consenting male neonates. Increasingly, adult American women undergo a wide variety of surgical interventions, some with considerable risk of complications, all in the name of "beauty" and the feminine ideal. So far, the World Health Organization and the United Nations have not elected to object to these American cultural practices as barbarous. A bioethicist with any sense of irony, however, might feel ill at ease in trying to explain why such "cosmetic" practices should be permitted to continue while female genital mutilation is everywhere condemned.[20]

Sandra Lane and Robert Rubenstein, writing more than a decade ago, suggested that the most ethical response to female genital mutilation among Westerners is to make common cause with women's groups in the affected nations that are trying to oppose the practice, but to allow those groups to take the lead in determining when, where, and how to register opposition.[21]

More recently, Ellen Gruenbaum cites TOSTAN, a Senegalese nongovernmental organization that encourages women's empowerment, as an example of such an approach.[22] Perhaps the most encouraging finding with regard to female genital mutilation is that its incidence appears inversely related to the level of education of the female population.[23] Possibly the most effective, and yet culturally respectful way that Western bioethics can help to eliminate this practice is to do everything possible to encourage female education in all developing nations.[24]


**::** Another Case Study: International Research Ethics

Disputes over HIV/AIDS research trials in Africa and Asia in the mid-1990s ushered in an era of renewed attention to the international dimensions of the ethics of research on human subjects. To critics of the HIV trials, the story was all too familiar. The United States government was sponsoring trials of the use of an antiretroviral drug AZT during pregnancy to prevent the transmission of HIV from the infected mother to the newborn. The current standard of care in the United States was to administer AZT to pregnant women according to an accepted dosage protocol. As the cost of treatment according to this protocol was extremely expensive for health authorities in developing countries, the trials were designed to test the efficacy of a lower-dose, shorter protocol that it was thought would be more affordable in those settings. The shorter protocol was compared to the standard U.S. protocol and also—hence the controversy—to a placebo control.

The use of a placebo control group was defended by the trial advocates on several grounds. The first ground was, in hindsight, not a defense so much as an admission of unethical conduct. Defenders noted that the current standard practice in those countries was to give no drug at all to pregnant HIV-positive women, so the placebo groups were not disadvantaged relative to the other members of their local communities. This so-called defense is a non-starter because it would justify virtually any exploitation of human subjects in the name of research, as long as one could find a society in which the average citizen was sufficiently deprived of decent care or actively mistreated.

Somewhat better defenses of the trials were, first, that host-country institutional research review boards (IRBs) had approved the trials, and that telling these boards that they did not understand the ethical treatment of human subjects in their own nations amounted itself to a sort of ethical imperialism; and second, that there was a legitimate need for a placebo control group in a society where, unlike the U.S., malnutrition and parasitic diseases were common, so that women receiving AZT in any dose might actually end up doing much worse than expected.[25]

The trials' critics sensed a depressing resemblance with a famous American study in which proven effective treatment for a sexually transmitted disease was withheld from people of color in a government-funded trial—the infamous Tuskegee syphilis study.[26] The facts that the Tuskegee study was designed specifically to be a study of the natural history of untreated disease, that effective treatment was withheld over a 40-year period from all study participants, and not merely from one group, and that no informed consent was obtained (and that to the contrary, subjects were actively lied to about the nature of the study), were all apparently passed over as irrelevant.[27]

In some ways, the most important rebuttal to the ethics of the AZT trials only came some years later. When the newer AIDS drugs, protease inhibitors, were introduced, proving dramatically superior to AZT in reducing viral load and reversing the symptoms of AIDS, their cost initially put them completely out of reach for most citizens of sub-Saharan Africa, the largest global reservoir of human HIV infection. The high cost of these drugs was initially addressed by many international health policy experts as an unfortunate but unalterable fact of life, and calls went forward for all HIV programs in Africa to stress prevention but to ignore treatment. A group of activists, however, believed that the high cost of these drugs represented, not a law of nature, but profiteering on the part of the global pharmaceutical industry. After a variety of actions, in which the U.S. government initially sided with the drug companies against the patients in need, the long-term result was a drastic reduction in the cost of anti-HIV drugs, making treatment a real possibility for patients in developing countries—though such treatment is unfortunately far from universal today.[28] The experience with protease inhibitors seemed to provide an object lesson relevant to the old AZT trials. If the problem is the high cost of drugs in developing countries, perhaps the answer is to attack that problem head on, rather than to conduct potentially exploitive research trials designed to see if people in those countries cannot somehow get by on a second-rate drug regimen.[29] Alternatively, if a cheaper drug regimen is just as good, it seems equally important that this fact be known in the developed world; so why not do the necessary research in the wealthier countries?

Given all of this, what are we to think today about the ethics of research in the developing world, especially when a developed country such as the United States sponsors the research (either via governmental agencies or via private foundations or corporations)? The quick answer to this question is that all problems have been resolved by requiring that these research trials conform to the ethical requirements that the National Institutes of Health and other U.S. agencies require for studies conducted in America; and that moreover, every nation who wishes to participate in any NIH-funded trial is required to replicate within its borders the same general sort of IRB system that operates in the United States. The U.S. government has expended considerable resources in training scientists and regulators in developing nations in how to institute and manage such an IRB system.

Patricia Marshall and Barbara Koenig see dangers in this approach. They begin with the assumption that it is not self-evident that U.S.

ethics are "right" for all nations, and that there may be specific local circumstances or social and cultural practices that deserve ethical respect even though they differ from the U.S. standard. They then suggest that the ideal framework for international research ethics would be much more the product of dialogue and consensus between the developed and the developing nations.

Such a consensus process is threatened by a number of factors. First, as Western thought is easily confused with modernity in developing countries, it may be very hard for local leaders to challenge or question the NIH ethical rules, however ill suited they may be to local conditions. Second, and worse, it is not as if the developing country is given any real choice here. Either they play the game by NIH rules, or they say goodbye to any hope of funding from that source—which could be make-or-break funding for the scientific careers of would-be local investigators, and all that might keep the most promising scientific talent from emigrating to the West. Even if we could determine with confidence that the NIH and American ethical standards are correct in every detail, it would still remain the case that thoughtful people in developing countries would believe that they were coerced into following those rules, not because they were ethically superior, but simply because the NIH held all the cards. Finally, Marshall and Koenig note the considerable drain on local resources required to mount and maintain a U.S.-style IRB program—a problem that is sadly not unique to the developing world and that commonly afflicts U.S. academic centers, too.[30]

The arguments raised by Marshall and Koenig cast considerable doubt on the wisdom of the current requirements that research ethics in the developing world simply ought to be a carbon copy of U.S. research ethics regulations. They omit, however, perhaps the most telling argument. At the same time that we are exporting the U.S. IRB system as the exemplar of everything that is ethical in research, thoughtful observers are more and more disillusioned with that system's current status.[31] To briefly summarize a debate that would take much more space to develop, IRBs are often attacked as being little more than consent-form editing bodies; and even after they are done editing the consent form, the result is a document that no American who lacks a graduate-school–level education can possibly read with comprehension. U.S. IRBs focus on the consent form to the exclusion of all the other aspects of the study design and study process that might harm or exploit subjects. Finally, as I argued in Chapter 1, the IRB system has dramatically failed in what should have been one of its prime goals—to persuade and educate U.S. investigators that good ethical thinking is part and parcel of good study design. U.S. clinical ethics has largely succeeded since the 1970s in educating clinicians on the basic concepts and vocabulary of clinical ethics, so that it would be indeed odd to find a physician who was completely unfamiliar with the notion of respect for patient autonomy. By contrast, it is still relatively common to find an investigator who believes that the only purpose of an IRB is to slow down, and create hassles for, the progress of research, and that the only possible relationship between the scientist and the IRB is an adversarial one.[32]

In short, it is sad if U.S. research ethics might not apply, or might apply best with considerable modifications, in developing countries, and yet this ethics is nonetheless forced upon those countries' research establishments. But it is even sadder if the United States continues to forge ahead with an inherently flawed system of research ethics regulation, when open dialogue with the international community might reveal alternative approaches from which U.S. ethicists and regulators might learn.[33]

A few years ago I was able to play a small role in the design of a project that seems to me to hold greater promise for addressing issues in international research ethics. The Center for Ethics and Humanities in the Life Sciences at Michigan State University partnered with the University of Malawi College of Medicine in a project supported by the NIH Fogarty International Center. The project selects scholars from sub-Saharan Africa and brings them to Michigan State University for one semester of course work. They then return to Africa where they receive additional academic training and undertake to complete a research project on African research ethics, under the guidance of two mentors, one from Africa and one from the United States.[34]

The goal of this project is assuredly *not* to indoctrinate Africans in the unthinking acceptance of the U.S. IRB system or any American system of research ethics. Rather it is to educate a cadre of Africans capable of original scholarly investigation of research ethics in Africa, and bringing both American and African ethical systems to bear on the problems that they identify. One might hope in the end that the U.S. scholars and mentors involved with the project will learn as many new ideas that might help to reform and advance research ethics in the U.S. as the African trainees learn from us.

NOTES TO CHAPTER 7

1. See table, Chapter 1, and associated text.
2. Marshall P. Koenig B. Accounting for culture in a globalized bioethics. *J Law Med Ethics* 32:252–66, 2004.

3. Goldenberg MJ. On evidence and evidence-based medicine: lessons from the philosophy of science. *Soc Sci Med* 62: 2621–32, 2006, quote on p. 2625. Goldenberg in turn quotes from Haraway D. Modest witness: feminist diffractions in science studies. In: Galison P, Stump D (eds.) *The disunity of science: boundaries, contexts, and power.* Stanford, CA: Stanford University Press, 1996, pp. 428–42, quote on p. 429.

4. Gillon R. Medical ethics: four principles plus attention to scope. *BMJ* 309:184–8, 1994.

5. Gillon R. Medical ethics: four principles plus attention to scope.

6. Tangwa GB. The traditional African perception of a person. Some implications for bioethics. *Hastings Cent Rep* 30(5):39–43, 2000.

7. Gillon's concerns are probably similar to those of Ruth Macklin, as analyzed by bioethicist-anthropologists Patricia Marshall and Barbara Koenig. The latter note that Macklin, in her extensive monograph opposing ethical relativism, makes a vigorous case for universally shared ethical principles. She seems to back off somewhat, however, when faced with the specific example of Navajo society and its members' belief in the power of words, making it an act of extreme disrespect for a physician to tell the patient the truth about a poor prognosis; in effect, this physician seems to the patient to be placing a hex on him. Macklin admits that in this setting, her "universal" rules about truthful disclosure and informed consent need to be modified; and she admits that this opens her up to a charge of ethical relativism. She defends herself against the charge by insisting that she is merely adopting reasonable flexibility in her application of the rules, and that the rules still reflect a more important, underlying ethical principle. Marshall and Koenig note that Macklin refuses to draw the lesson that they believe to be correct, that "morality is culturally embedded"; Marshall P, Koenig B. Accounting for culture in a globalized bioethics. *J Law Med Ethics* 32:252–66, 2004, quote on p. 260. They in turn are citing Macklin R. *Against relativism: cultural diversity and the search for ethical universals in medicine.* New York: Oxford University Press, 1999. I contend below, in the section on relativism, that from the fact that morality is culturally embedded, it does not follow that we lack a perspective outside of any given culture to criticize the ethics of that culture's beliefs and practices.

8. Rorty R. Pragmatism, relativism, and irrationalism. In: *Consequences of pragmatism.* Minneapolis: University of Minnesota Press, 1982, pp. 160–75.

9. Walker MU. *Moral understandings: a feminist study in ethics.* New York: Routledge, 1998, pp. 7–9, 29–46.

10. Kopelman LM. The incompatibility of the United Nations' goals and conventionalist ethical relativism. *Developing World Bioethics* 5:234–43, 2005.

11. Nussbaum MC. *Frontiers of justice: disability, nationality, species membership.* Cambridge, MA: Belknap/Harvard University Press, 2006, pp. 255–62.

12. The terminology is notoriously controversial. Some would require that we adopt a culturally neutral term, such as "female genital cutting," to avoid the prejudgment that is associated with the term "mutilation." I have

adopted the more judgmental language of "mutilation" because that term has been officially adopted by the United Nations and the World Health Organization; see, for example, Braddy CM, Files JA. Female genital mutilation: cultural awareness and clinical considerations. *J Midwifery Womens Health* 52:158–63, 2007.

13. On the complexity of the practice, see, for example, Lane SD, Rubenstein RA. Judging the other: responding to traditional female genital surgeries. *Hastings Cent Rep* 26(3):31–40, 1996; Baron EM, Denmark FL. An exploration of female genital mutilation. *Ann NY Acad Sci* 1087:339–55, 2006; Gruenbaum E. Socio-cultural dynamics of female genital cutting: research findings, gaps, and directions. *Cult Health Sex* 7:429–41, 2005. Baron and Denmark cite a 2005 UNICEF study that indicates that as many as 80 percent of African women aged 15–49 support continuation of the practice. Naturally, a majority of women endorsing a practice that primarily affects women does not necessarily give one grounds to favor it, since the women's opinions might represent not optimal free choice, but rather false consciousness or a reflection of the severely constrained choices available to them in society.

14. "Negotiations on the ratification of the Protocol of the African charter on the rights of women in Africa," http://www.stopfgmc.org/client/sheet.aspx?root=256&sheet=1721&lang=en-US (accessed April 22, 2007).

15. For an instance of increasing frequency of female genital mutilation among some communities in Sudan, see Gruenbaum E. Socio-cultural dynamics of female genital cutting: research findings, gaps, and directions. *Cult Health Sex* 7:429–41, 2005, particularly p. 433.

16. This list is summarized from Baron EM, Denmark FL. An exploration of female genital mutilation. *Ann NY Acad Sci* 1087:339–55, 2006.

17. This statement is true primarily of Type 1 and Type 2 circumcision (less extreme) according to the WHO classification, and of practices performed in older, near-puberty females.

18. This statement is true primarily of Type 3 (infibulation), the most extreme form, which reportedly is used in only about 15 percent of all cases; Baron EM, Denmark FL. An exploration of female genital mutilation. *Ann NY Acad Sci* 1087:339–55, 2006.

19. "Erroneously" here assumes that the only legitimate religious teaching occurs centrally, as when, for example, the Koran dictates the entirety of Islamic teaching. At the community level, numerous *fatwas* by local clerics can be cited in defense of female genital mutilation; Baron EM, Denmark FL. An exploration of female genital mutilation. *Ann NY Acad Sci* 1087:339–55, 2006.

20. Conroy AM. Female genital mutilation: whose problem, whose solution? *BMJ* 333:106–7, 2006.

21. Lane SD, Rubenstein RA. Judging the other: responding to traditional female genital surgeries. *Hastings Cent Rep* 26(3):31–40, 1996.

22. Gruenbaum E. Socio-cultural dynamics of female genital cutting: research findings, gaps, and directions. *Cult Health Sex* 7:429–41, 2005.

23. Baron EM, Denmark FL. An exploration of female genital mutilation. *Ann NY Acad Sci* 1087:339–55, 2006.
24. See Chapter 10 for more on obligations that wealthier nations owe to poor ones.
25. Gambia Government/Medical Research Council Joint Ethical Committee. Ethical issues facing medical research in developing countries. *Lancet* 351:286–7, 1998.
26. Lurie P, Wolfe SM. Unethical trials of interventions to reduce perinatal transmission of the human immunodeficiency virus in developing countries. *N Engl J Med* 337:853–6, 1997; Angell M. The ethics of research in the Third World. *N Engl J Med* 337:847–9, 1997.
27. One might respond that for the infants who contracted HIV from their mothers because their mothers received no antiretroviral treatment, it hardly mattered whether the treatment was withheld for 40 years or 40 days, or whether only one group of subjects as opposed to all the subjects were so deprived. Moreover, there were allegations that the actual consent process in the communities in Africa and Asia left many illiterate subjects still in the dark about what the study actually consisted of, and whether or not all would receive treatment.
28. Bond P. Globalization, pharmaceutical pricing, and South African health policy: managing confrontation with U.S. firms and politicians. *Int J Health Serv* 29:765–92, 1999; Barnard D. In the high court of South Africa, case number 4138/98: the global politics of access to low-cost AIDS drugs in poor countries. *Kennedy Inst Ethics J* 12:159–74, 2002.
29. I say here potentially *exploitive* research trials because I would argue that a non-exploitation standard is the correct one for research ethics, no matter where in the world the trial is conducted; see for example Miller FG, Brody H. A critique of clinical equipoise. Therapeutic misconception in the ethics of clinical trials. *Hastings Cent Rep* 33(3):19–28, 2003. This debate has important implications for international research ethics because, according to the position I would defend, the Declaration of Helsinki, officially the basis for research ethics around the world, is in fact flawed and incoherent by trying to reduce the ethics of research to the ethics of therapeutic medicine. I cannot here fully develop or defend that argument. See also Emanuel EJ, Wendler D, Killen J, et al. What makes clinical research ethical in developing countries ethical? The benchmarks of ethical research. *J Infect Dis* 189:930–7, 2004.
30. Marshall P, Koenig B. Accounting for culture in a globalized bioethics. *J Law Med Ethics* 32:252–66, 2004.
31. United States National Bioethics Advisory Commission. *Ethical and policy issues in research involving human participants.* Bethesda, MD: National Bioethics Advisory Commission, 2001; Vanderpool HY. Introduction and overview: Ethics, historical case studies, and the research enterprise. In: Vanderpool HY, ed. *The ethics of research involving human subjects: facing the twenty-first century.* Frederick, MD: University Publishing Group, 1996, pp. 1–30; Miller FG. Revisiting the Belmont Report: the ethical significance

of the distinction between clinical research and medical care. *APA Newsletter on Philosophy and Medicine* 5(2):10–14, 2005.

32. Do researchers learn to practice misbehavior? [anonymous letter to editor]. *Hastings Cent Rep* 36(2):4, 2006.

33. It is important to note that the current IRB system in the U.S. was basically put in place in the late 1970s in response to the ethical principles laid out in the Belmont Report. I agree with Miller that there is little reason to dispute the Belmont foundation, at least within the U.S. society and culture; Miller FG. Revisiting the Belmont Report: the ethical significance of the distinction between clinical research and medical care. *APA Newsletter on Philosophy and Medicine* 5(2):10–14, 2005. But the IRB regulatory system is basically a bureaucracy that was created (as was the Belmont Report itself) in response to specific scandals in research ethics that came to attention during the 1960s and 1970s, and that were especially highlighted by the lack of adequate informed consent. It would be indeed odd if such a system had not gotten creaky in the joints after about thirty years and was not in need of an upgrade. Such a need would hardly be an embarrassment to the thoughtful, well-intentioned people who first designed the system and then have more recently been doing their best to make it work.

34. For details, see http://www.bioethics.msu.edu/pages/intnat/index.html (accessed November 18, 2007). I am grateful to Tom Tomlinson, Elizabeth Bogdan-Lovis, Joseph Mfutso-Bengo, Paul Ndebele, and others involved in the project for the ideas here described.

# 8 ::

# Race and Health Disparities

It seems that a majority of U.S. bioethicists support substantial health-care reform, buying into the argument that it is immoral for a country as rich as ours to deny such a large percentage of the population guaranteed access to routine, basic health care.[1] When we ask why bioethics has not succeeded in persuading the majority of the American public of this moral truth, the reply often given is that Americans have been unwilling to support major-health care reform because it is seen as a large government entitlement program, which we tend to view with extreme suspicion. In turn, it is said, Americans oppose such entitlement programs out of convictions that these programs are inefficient and ineffective, are prone to waste and abuse, and would undermine individuals' taking responsibility for themselves as they ought.

In April, 2007, Eduardo Porter wrote a *New York Times* article based on interviews with a number of prominent economists and social scientists. He concluded that these stated reasons to oppose government spending programs often hid a deeper reason. Americans might be much more willing to vote in favor of such programs—provided that people *like themselves* were the beneficiaries. The greater the racial and ethnic diversity of the community, and the more likely it is that voters see their tax dollars going to assist "the other," the lower the support for any spending, be it for health care, schools, or welfare.[2]

In sum, one of the reasons why the United States has not yet done the ethically correct thing with regard to health care access for all might be racism. If "racism" sounds overly harsh in the present context,

I would simply note that by that word, I do not mean solely the *conscious* dislike of or wish to treat badly people of any given racial group. I would include under the title both unconscious individual habits of thought and ingrained social practices that have the result of seriously limiting the life opportunities of members of that racial group. A society, that is, can be racist even if no individual member of that society harbors any malicious intent.

Porter's observation is important particularly in the light of political developments in the United States in recent years. There is a growing movement to reject affirmative action, in legislatures, courts, and in public referenda. There have been a number of reasons for this rejection, and some arguing for the rejection are members of minority groups who have previously been favored by affirmative action measures. But I believe that one widespread reason to oppose affirmative action today is the belief that the form and degree of racial discrimination that made affirmative action programs seem justified when they were first introduced some decades ago have faded into the past. Today, its opponents claim, affirmative action no longer serves as a corrective to unjust discrimination, and it has become in itself a form of unjust discrimination—so therefore we ought to oppose it.

I believe that this reasoning is both wrong and dangerous. The research that Eduardo Porter reviewed suggests that racism is alive and well in the American body politic. Does this, however, make racial and ethnic concerns a fit subject for bioethical inquiry?

In the remainder of this chapter I will address primarily concerns about race, and use African-Americans as the focus of most of the discussion. I believe that a careful analysis will show that if one were to engage in a similar inquiry about "ethnicity," one would see the concerns there closely tracking the discussion about "race."

## ∷ Is There a Distinct African-American Bioethics?

One theoretical way to flesh out a call for the study of racial and ethnic concerns in bioethics is to propose that there are in fact unique strains or types of bioethics—an African-American bioethics, a Hispanic bioethics, and so forth. This would seem quite consistent with a model we encountered at the start of the last chapter, when it was asserted that there might be such a thing as a uniquely African bioethics. Is such an approach plausible?[3]

The philosopher Jorge L.A. Garcia has offered a catalogue of the features that an distinctively African-American bioethics would possess. He suggests that such a bioethics would be:

- anti-majoritarian and anti-utilitarian
- anti-situationalist
- distrustful of an "ethics of trust"
- focused on the patient as the one with the decision to make
- sympathetic toward families without romanticizing them
- free from the bonds of scientism
- open to insights from religious faith
- not beholden to a neutralist political liberalism (which, in Garcia's view, is often antireligious)[4]

Garcia proceeds to offer explanations of each of these features, highlighting ways in which the experience of African-Americans in the United States would reasonably lead them toward acceptance of a bioethics or philosophy of this sort, and of a rejection of a philosophical viewpoint with the opposite features.[5]

Garcia's further comments seem to me to be apt:

> So conceived, everyone can and should learn from medical ethical reflection that is duly informed by consideration of experiences widespread among African Americans. Indeed, the chief importance of such an ethical perspective—that is, an approach duly informed by reflection on African-American lives—is not as something self-sufficient but rather lies in what it can contribute to an overall view that takes cognizance of, and remains faithful to, a variety of such points of view. This and other particular perspectives matter chiefly as vantage points that yield vital input, but are ultimately to be transcended by their incorporation into a comprehensive moral vision.[6]

I take this to suggest that we need not trouble ourselves with questions about whether there is a *distinctive* African-American bioethics, or indeed exactly what that claim might entail; or whether there are *essential* features of the African-American experience that give rise to such a bioethics. For our purposes it is enough to claim that a bioethics that is "duly informed by considerations of experiences widespread" within an important racial or ethnic group is likely to be a bioethics that is thereby enriched and deepened.

One might object: on what basis can we say that African-Americans are anti-utilitarian? Does it not seem more probable that it is simply the case that Garcia himself doesn't like utilitarianism? But this misses the main point. Can Garcia demonstrate a plausible connection between some *widespread* element of the African-American experience and an anti-utilitarian viewpoint? After reading his analysis, will we be inclined to say, "I can see now how people who have been through that sort of experience might well feel that way about utilitarianism"? If so, then he has deepened our understanding of bioethics to that degree, and I see no reason to demand more.

## ⠃⠃ What Is Race?

Today's medical literature on race seems conflicted if not self-contradictory. For instance, one body of literature proclaims that the recent discoveries regarding the human genome ought to put the lid on any appeals to race as a useful concept in medicine. There simply cannot be any genetic basis for that construct we call "race." At the same time, articles continue to appear in medical journals that report the different rates at which various diseases, or responses to treatments, occur in different racial groups. It would certainly seem difficult to understand why such articles are either written or published, if the concept of race is medically useless. To further mystify us, yet another group of genomic scientists reports the results of haplotype mapping, telling us of important genetic differences that arise among "Europeans," "Africans," and "Japanese," for instance.[7]

If the medical literature seems confused, other bodies of work seem even more so. What are we to make, for example, of the current use of the term "color-blind" in discussions of social policy? At one point in recent history, this term would have been used by those, probably to the left of the political spectrum, who objected to unjust discrimination against people of color, and who demanded that the state take action to correct these injustices. Today, we are more likely to find this term used by those more to the right, who object whenever the state utilizes racial identifiers, even if the goal is to prevent or to provide restitution for unjust discrimination.[8] To take one medical example, some have urged that public health agencies be prohibited from using any racially identified information, so that it would become impossible, in effect, to determine whether racial disparities exist in health or in health-care services.[9]

Whatever one thinks of the rightness or wrongness of any of these conclusions, we must address the prior question of whether people are actually talking about the same thing. Here, the skills of philosophical bioethics would appear to be useful. By analogy, Bruce Miller argued a quarter-century ago that some of the debates on patient autonomy were in fact pointless, because people were not arguing about the same thing when they used the word "autonomy." He proposed four distinct senses of "autonomy," and thereby considerably aided further analysis and discussion.[10] Miller's study remains an excellent model of how theoretical clarification in ethics can yield valuable practical outcomes.

Following Miller's example, I would propose that there are four relevant senses of "race" currently at work in medical, bioethical, and public policy debates. The four senses in turn can be subdivided depending on whether the construct is seen as predominantly a biological fact about the human organism, or as a social construction, as in Table 8.1.[11]

Classic race is the historic view of race that recent medical and genomic science has thoroughly discredited. On this view, inherited superficial characteristics such as skin color, shape of the head and eyes, and so forth, are correlated with much deeper and more significant inherited differences that naturally divide the human race into a relatively few subtypes. Therefore, by observing the superficial appearance of an individual, one can draw scientifically valid conclusions about the sorts of diseases that person is likely to develop, intelligence and character traits, and a wide variety of other important aspects of life.

To be a bit clearer, no one denies that there are superficial characteristics such as skin color, facial features, hair texture, and the like that tend to cluster in groups and that are inherited. Where classic race concepts erred, by our analysis, is imagining that somehow these superficial differences were a sign of something that went "all the way down." It was thought that by inspecting the outside of an individual, one could reasonably infer a long list of other characteristics about that individual, including susceptibilities to different diseases as well as intelligence and character traits. I will assume that all discussants agree that this view of human biology is no longer tenable.

TABLE 8.1. Four Senses of "Race"

| Race | | | |
|---|---|---|---|
| Biological Variable | | Social Construction | |
| Classic | Geographic | Self-ascribed | Other-ascribed |

Geographic race might be viewed as genomic science's effort to retrieve a baby, once science has discarded the bathwater of classic race. Geographic race starts from the assumption, reasonable on its face, that humans were over many generations most likely to mate with, and hence share genetic material with, those who were geographically close to them. Therefore, even if we cannot divide the human race into distinct "races" according to the classic-race theory, we ought to expect to find a variety of genetic traits clustering according to a population's continent of origin. If some of the superficial appearances we call "racial" today correlate reasonably well with one's continent of origin, then we would expect those appearances to serve as helpful, even if only rough proxies for the associated genetic clusters.

I do not have space here for a detailed critique of geographic race, but I would suggest that we regard this category with considerable suspicion, as it is likely to collapse back into one or more of the other senses of "race." It may collapse back into classic race because the assumptions attached to that long-dominant biological theory may not have been sufficiently scrubbed from the methodology used by today's genomic scientists, despite their conscious efforts to jettison that baggage. It may collapse back into one or both of the social-construction sense of "race" because we can only detect genetic clusters when we sample a given population of individuals. If these individuals were labeled as "Japanese" or "European" or "African" because of either self-ascribed or other-ascribed racial labels, then one cannot separate the resultant genetic clusterings from the socially constructed assumptions used to gather the initial data. Or, to put it another way, we have simply relocated all the ambiguity and confusion that used to be associated with the term "race" to the term "population."[12]

The two social-construction senses of race are distinct and yet mutually influential. They are distinct because a person may be labeled differently by the two routes of ascription. It has been shown that a substantial number of people seem to have changed their race between the issuance of their birth and death certificates, and a case has been reported of a person who had three different racial labels affixed within the confines of a single medical record.[13] The race that appears on one's birth certificate of course represents other-ascribed race, while the race listed on a death certificate is much more likely to reflect self-ascribed race. Self-ascribed race may appear in one portion of the hospital chart (perhaps with the admitting demographic information) while other-ascribed race appears elsewhere (such as the physician's history and physical exam).

On the other hand, the two social-construction senses of race are mutually influential because very commonly, what we think of ourselves is shaped and altered by what those around us think of us. There are, for instance, many U.S. immigrants from Caribbean islands or South American nations who today regard themselves as black, even though while they were growing up in their countries of origin, there was no such category in evidence that they were aware of.

With this brief discussion, we can begin to see how specifying the sense of "race" that is in play may prevent serious practical misunderstandings. What does it mean, for instance, to say that the incidence of a certain disease varies among racial groups? One might be making a biological claim that these groups represent populations who originated in distinct continents, and who ended up with distinct genetic traits that made them more susceptible to the disease (geographic race). Alternatively, one may be making a claim that one's social status influences the sorts of diseases one is prone to, and racial categories are an important part of that social status (other-ascribed race).

What are we, for a further example, to make of the proposal that racial identifiers be eliminated from public health data? The advocate of this proposal may justify it based on the fact that race has been discredited as a medical category. This, of course, applies only to classic race (though I would argue that geographic race is also suspect). Self-ascribed and other-ascribed race are social constructions, and it seems a legitimate goal of public health inquiry to determine whether differences in social status influence one's state of health. Therefore, objecting to racial identifiers in health data is revealed as a form of category mistake.[14]

Perhaps this suggested analysis of the various senses of "race" is simply wrong, or perhaps it needs further refinement and development. My point is less to argue for it and more to suggest that there is important philosophical work to be done regarding the concept of "race" in a variety of discourses today. It would seem to be within the realm of bioethics to do that work.

## ∷ Whiteness

Soraya Sarhaddi Nelson, a National Public Radio correspondent covering Afghanistan, was interviewed for NPR's *Morning Edition* during a return visit to the United States. She described the contrast between

Kabul, where Western customs were generally accepted, and smaller Afghan towns, where she might have to don a burka lest she become a victim of violence. The experience of working in Afghanistan, she added, forced her to become much more aware of being a woman, and she found the attention that she had to pay to her gender very tiring.[15]

One might imagine an American male reporter, similarly assigned to Afghanistan. He would face many differences between life there and back home. But he would not be confronted personally with issues regarding being a male, and being male would not expose him to any particular risks or inconveniences in Afghanistan. If he were an unimaginative type, he might even dismiss the complaints of his female colleagues, wondering whether they were seeking undeserved sympathy or privileges by insisting that some *special* liability attached to their femaleness.

It is, however, unlikely that the hypothetical male reporter would be this obtuse. He would have in common with the women the fact that he was used to American ways and that Afghan customs were quite different. But what if the conditions that created special problems for the women, but not for the men, were part of the background conditions of life in America, and had been there as long as the man had lived? Would he then be perceptive enough to notice?

I have used this extended analogy to back into the concept of "whiteness." The term is problematic because there is, I gather, a certain amount of academic smugness that has become associated with it—associations with terms such as "postmodern," "postcolonial," and "problematizing."[16] I will try therefore to express the core idea of "whiteness," as I understand it, in as straightforward a way as possible.

"Whiteness" refers to the way we form an implicit image of what is normal, what is good, and what is valued, and then adopt that vantage point without realizing and accepting that we have done so. At the same time, we very explicitly label all portions of the world, and all people, who do not conform to the normative model. If we say directly, "white people are better than black people," we naturally arouse the question of why this is so, and whether such a posture is consistent with ethical principles of justice and equity. Yet these same ethical questions are swept under the carpet if the white people become invisible in their whiteness, while the black people stand out boldly in their blackness. It then seems simply an objective fact about the world that being black is something that has to be discussed, argued about, dissected; while being white is a "natural" way of being that requires no defense or explanation.

Leonard Pitts, Jr., the Pulitzer-Prize–winning black columnist, commented on one manifestation of "whiteness." He received a spate of e-mails when it was revealed that a black athlete, Michael Vick, had been involved in an illegal dog-fighting ring. The e-mails came from white readers and, as Pitts summarized, asked why he did not "lay into this individual the way you 'always' do white guys." Pitts correctly observed that this query had very little to do with Michael Vick; and it had little to do with the many other black public figures that Pitts had in fact skewered in earlier columns, in his inimitable fashion. Rather, he wrote, the issue was, "that some white people—emphasize, *some*—seem to feel that they have a perfect right to demand, overtly and repeatedly, that a black professional prove himself to them."[17] Such demands that one constantly prove one's basic right just to be there and do one's job can be extremely taxing and fatiguing, as well as depressing and demoralizing, to an extent that someone who never is subjected to such demands probably cannot appreciate.

What turns invisible on this account is not so much "whiteness" as "white privilege." A culture that stresses individual responsibility, and in which white privilege has been rendered invisible, assumes that when white people succeed in life, it must be because they worked hard, developed their talents diligently, and in general personally earned everything that they received. Since white privilege is invisible, the extent to which their success depended on the good luck of having been born white becomes invisible as well. The social "norm," then, becomes that everyone can succeed if only they work hard and act responsibly. If black people do not succeed to the same degree that white people do, the obvious answer is that they must be lazy, or perhaps that they are genetically inferior and lack important talents. The white people's success "proves" that the blacks could have succeeded too if only they had tried harder. Such a view seems to be lurking behind the nasty e-mails that columnist Leonard Pitts received—that if a white person has a newspaper column, it must be because he is a good writer and has interesting things to say; if a black person has a column, it must mean that he is incompetent but that some bumbling liberal lets him write the column anyway, as an exercise in "political correctness" or "liberal guilt."

I grew up in a family where it was generally accepted as a given that I would attend and graduate from college. Many of my older relatives were college graduates, some with advanced degrees, and could give me practical advice on college applications and related matters.

I attended a high school where, even though only a minority of the graduates attended college, the college-bound students were looked up to and respected. I never had to deal with a peer group that regarded me as some sort of traitor to their cause because I sought to go to college and succeed in an academic life. As a result of my upbringing, I have very limited ability to imagine what it is like to attend college and to graduate when one is the first in one's family to do so; when no close friends or relatives can give one any advice on how to do this; and when the entire message conveyed by one's previous schooling is that college is out of bounds for one to aspire to. I can look at a person coming from such a background, who somehow did manage both to attend and to complete college, and see that she earned a bachelor's degree. What I cannot see is the sheer amount of *extra* energy that that person had to expend, both to do all the work required to study for exams and to make good grades, *and also* to overcome all those persistent barriers to success.

A good example of the invisibility of whiteness occurred in the time following the September 11, 2001, terrorist attacks. Islamic leaders in the United States, hoping to head off discrimination against their community, stressed the peaceful nature of Islamic religious teachings and the community's lack of support for, and repugnance at, the activities of terrorists. Whenever another Islamic terrorist outrage occurred, these leaders were castigated if they did not immediately and explicitly disown and condemn the perpetrators. Those "white" Americans who castigated the Islamic leaders (perhaps the same crowd that sent the nasty e-mails to Pitts) never saw any irony in the fact that none of them felt any responsibility to disown the act of a white American who committed a heinous crime. When a white person does something terrible, he and he alone did it; when a member of a minority group does something wrong, "one of them" did it. This is just another way of saying that American Muslims, especially in the wake of 9/11, ceased to be white.

Catherine Myser, discussing the importance of whiteness for bioethics, quotes James Baldwin: "[no] one was white before he/she came to America. It took generations, and a vast amount of coercion. . . . White men—from Norway, for example, where they were Norwegians—became white . . . and we—who were not Black before we got here either, were defined as Black by the slave trade."[18] I take Baldwin to mean that we like to imagine that "white" and "black" are natural types. We discover them by observing the world as it is. It is a simple fact of human biology that white people pretty much lack melanin in their skin and black people have a good deal of it. But in fact, white and black (in the relevant senses) have nothing to do with melanin and biology, and everything to do with relationships of dominance and power. White and black are defined through social relationships. Baldwin's observation is still factually true. As I previously noted, people from many societies move to the United States and suddenly discover that they are regarded as black people, when in their countries of origin, there is really no category corresponding to "black" comparable to the United States. These people *become* black by coming to America. Other societies besides ours may have their own problems with racism and racial categories; but the peculiar way we define and deal with "blackness" seems uniquely ours.

Why is whiteness of interest to bioethics? In a narrow sense, it helps us understand some important debates around race relationships, such as today's attacks on affirmative action, in which it is argued that any affirmative action program today would amount to giving unjust privileges to members of minority groups. We can now better understand how the persistent privileges associated with whiteness can be so invisible to people who argue this way. Affirmative action is of importance in bioethics because of the question of what racial and ethnic mix ought to be present in a medical school class (for example) if the resulting physician workforce is to be best suited to meet the medical care needs of a diverse population.

The importance of whiteness, however, goes far beyond affirmative action debates. It is an important insight for bioethics whenever we discover a pervasive and long-lived mechanism by which major ethical questions can effectively be hidden from view. In matters of race relationships, American society is like the husband who shows up for marital counseling and tells the therapist, "I'm fine, thank you very much; it's my wife who's crazy and who needs your help." We in America have a history of black problems, Hispanic problems, American Indian problems, but never any white problems. Bioethics must develop delicate antennae for any such strategy of denying ethically problematic power relationships.

## ⠴ The Ethical Status of Health Disparities

In 1993, Knox H. Todd and his colleagues studied the treatment of pain in an emergency department in Southern California. To assure that there could be no doubt that the patients studied had significant pain, they restricted the review to cases of long bone fractures clearly visible on x-rays. Normally, for such an event, a patient would be given a powerful narcotic analgesic such as morphine. The investigators found that patients with Hispanic-sounding surnames were about half as likely to get such a narcotic as other patients.[19] Reportedly, when the physicians in the department were told of these results, they were aghast. They had no awareness that they had been giving patients such starkly different treatment.

This study is emblematic of most of the now-extensive literature on racial and ethnic health disparities in the United States. It is relatively easy to find conditions for which either the treatment administered, or the health outcomes achieved, or both, are significantly deficient for patients from a minority group as compared with the white majority. The physicians responsible for the care of those patients are genuinely shocked and deny any conscious intent to provide a different level of care. After the disparities are pointed out, and remedial measures are instituted, a good deal of the time nothing changes.[20] Despite this overall depressing picture, there have been some instances of improvement.[21]

I am aware of little bioethics literature on the topic of health disparities. I believe that there are two reasons for this. First, the ethical issues relevant to health disparities appear to be shallow and uninteresting. If people are being discriminated against in health care on the basis of race, then that is wrong, pure and simple; one needs no in-depth ethical analysis. That in turn raises the question of whether people *are* being discriminated against; and that in turn requires an empirical assessment of what causes health disparities and what resolves them. Such inquiries can be extremely daunting and require skills quite different from how most bioethicists were trained. So it is not surprising if bioethics has decided that health disparities is best left to others to discuss.

To begin to see how bioethics might make a serious contribution to discussions of health disparities, I will suggest two general approaches. First, I will review some suggestions from Norman Daniels, the American philosopher who has probably contributed more than any other to discussions of the just allocation of health resources. Next, I will propose an approach that is less theoretically inclined and closer to the nitty-gritty empirical work.

## ⦂ Daniels's Approach to Disparities

Daniels addresses racial and class-related health disparities as part of a larger agenda, to extend bioethics' reach into questions of equity and population health.[22] Daniels has tended in his work to adopt a strongly theory-driven approach, and this is the way that he tackles the health disparities issue.

Daniels begins with the conflict between two approaches to population health. A health maximizer will favor policies that improve the overall health of the entire population as much as possible, regardless of how benefits are distributed within the population. A health egalitarian will seek to reduce inequalities and disparities within the population, even if the policies adopted fail to improve the overall health of the population as much as some alternative policies would. Daniels adds that the maximizing strategy may be favored over the egalitarian strategy by funders who want to see immediate, easily measurable return on investment.

One way that the health egalitarian can defend an anti-disparity policy against criticism from a health maximizer is to claim that a particular disparity arises from an inequity society has been responsible for in the past, at least to some degree. If we assume that today's racial inequalities are based at least in part on a history of socially sanctioned racism, our duty to make it a priority to resolve health disparities that affect black citizens can be based on the rough ethical equivalent of "we broke it, we fix it." The egalitarian should then expect the rejoinder from an opponent who seeks to reduce the extent to which past social policies are truly to blame for the present state of affairs. These rejoinders may range from crude victim-blaming to quite sophisticated invocations of multiple factors, as we will see below.

Daniels further justifies his more theoretical approach by pointing out certain paradoxes that can, he believes, ultimately be resolved only by a better theoretical understanding of health inequality and justice. One concrete example that he gives involves black and white infant mortality rates between 1954 and 1998. During this period, the racial disparity worsened; the black infant mortality rate was 64 percent higher than the white rate in 1954, and 130 percent higher in 1998. Nevertheless, during that interval, the infant mortality rates declined for both whites and blacks. Indeed they dropped more for blacks than for whites—by 20.8 deaths per thousand among whites and by 30.1 deaths per thousand among blacks. One way to look at these numbers would declare victory by pointing out that the black rate dropped more than the white rate, even though both improved. Another way is to declare a crisis by pointing to the widening gap between black and white infants. Daniels appears to argue that only through a clearer theoretical understanding of the relevant concepts of justice can we choose between these competing accounts.

Daniels summarizes by listing a set of contributions that he believes that bioethics can make with regard to health disparities:

1. advance the existing analyses of unresolved problems in distributive justice
2. clarify when a health inequality is in fact an injustice
3. explain the relationship between #1 and #2; that is, how the injustice affects or is related to the unresolved distributive problems
4. clarify what counts as a reasonable rate of progress toward reducing the identified health inequalities
5. test the implications of #1–#4 above for actual health–policy choices, such as the dissemination of new technologies
6. develop a general theory of a fair, legitimate process for resolving reasonable disagreements as to what policies should be followed
7. apply the theory developed in #6 to specific institutional and policy contexts[23]

It appears here that Daniels is calling for a largely theoretical body of work in contributions #1–#3. His #4–#5 then seem to descend to the level of practicalities and actual policy decisions. He admits that an ideal theory of justice will go only so far in resolving disagreements among policies—after the philosophical theorists have done their best, there will still remain unresolved matters about which reasonable onlookers can disagree. His response to that point, in #6, is once again to demand a theory—this time a procedural theory. I understand Daniels here to be calling for a more theoretical understanding of the issues that we addressed in Chapter 5, since I would assume that one or another of the models we discussed for community dialogue in bioethics might be the sort of democratic deliberation that Daniels would favor for resolving still-outstanding policy dilemmas.

## ⠶ An Alternative Approach to Disparities

Daniels's approach obviously offers some useful insights. Let me suggest, by contrast, an account of a bioethics agenda around health disparities that takes off from a more pragmatic point of departure, following step by step the process of empirical investigation that might identify health disparities and their causal factors.

*Data-gathering.* The first step in inquiry is data-gathering. One must be able to identify a disparity in either treatment rates or outcomes in order to know that some sort of inquiry is warranted. To the onlooker, this step seems completely straightforward, given the ability of health-service experts to provide us with the most arcane statistics seemingly at the drop of a hat.

Appearances, however, may be deceiving. Naturally, to identify disparities, one must know the racial or ethnic identity of any given patient in the population being studied. According to one recent survey, "Despite growing recognition of the need for accurate and timely data on race and ethnicity, the collection of this information is neither widely practiced nor accepted by the health care industry. No standard-ized requirements exist for the collection, categorization, or use of data on race and ethnicity."[24] A failure to appreciate the different senses of "race," as we have discussed, can prove a further barrier to standard-ized measurement approaches.

There are certainly important ethical issues related to gathering such data. The authors of the report go on to state that a model data-gathering policy should include "a mechanism for guaranteeing confi-dentiality and preventing misuse, as well as a communication strategy for addressing patients' concerns...."[25] Effective communication with the minority community is critically important, given Patricia King's ethical concerns about using racial identifiers in research generally. King would, I believe, in the end support health-disparities research. Yet she also points out the many ways in which research involving racial identifiers has historically been used to the detriment of the minority community, despite the promises and good intentions of the investiga-tors in many instances. She submits that the burden of justification must always be borne by those who would use such identifiers.[26]

King is concerned about gathering racially identified data because of concerns for the well-being of the minority community. Others, more recently, have voiced opposition to gathering racially identified data, on the grounds that it violates the goal of "color-blind" governmental pol-icies. This latter position that might at first seem similar to King's, but I believe it to be totally different in spirit as well as in consequence. What exactly would it mean to adopt as one's ideal that our government ought to be color-blind? To take the ideal seriously would require first of all an appreciation of the historical record that demonstrates how difficult that ideal will be to achieve. In light of that history, a true ded-ication to that ideal would appear to require that we carefully attend to interim measurements of progress or lack of progress. We would want to be very careful that our so-called "color-blindness" is truly having the desired, advantageous effect. By contrast, the failure to make these measurements, and especially any public policy that would render such measurement impossible, would seem to be strong evidence that one did not truly espouse the color-blind ideal after all. The person invoking the "color-blind" rhetoric is indeed blind, but rather to the fact that color still matters a great deal in our society, and that the people whose lives are being damaged by our attention to color are to be rendered socially invisible by this rhetoric.

*Causal ascription.* Suppose that we have completed the data-gathering and have discovered, let us say, that African-Americans die more frequently and at younger ages of congestive heart failure (CHF) than do white Americans. The next empirical step is to try to discern the causal factors behind this observation. Depending on what they might be, the implications for health policy may be vastly different.

The following is a no doubt incomplete, but perhaps representative list of the causal hypotheses that must be entertained as possible explanations for the health disparities data.

1. Blacks are genetically different from whites. The biochemical and cellular processes leading to CHF are different and respond differently to today's standard treatments. These differences are inherited in much the same way that the gene for sickle cell disease is inherited.
2. Blacks are at greater risk for CHF than whites due to lifestyle differences. For instance, hypertension is a major risk factor for CHF, and one of the things that put people at risk for hypertension is a high dietary salt intake. Because of cultural beliefs and practices, blacks routinely consume many more high-salt foods than do whites.
3. Blacks are at greater risk for CHF than whites due to lifestyle differences, but these differences have little or nothing to do with culture. For example, smoking may put one at greater risk for CHF, and more blacks than whites may smoke, though there is nothing in the "black culture" as such that encourages smoking.
4. Blacks and whites may be at equal biological risk for CHF. Whites simply receive better treatment than do blacks, and receive it more quickly, thus explaining the differential mortality rates. This in turn could occur because the same physicians treat both white and black patients, but employ different treatment strategies for

the two groups either for conscious or for unconscious reasons. Or it might occur because black and white patients seek care in different places. For example, blacks may receive their care in emergency departments where there is no follow-up and so receive a lesser quality care for a chronic condition such as CHF.

5. Blacks and whites are at equal "biological" risk for CHF and receive equivalent treatments once they develop the disease. But blacks are at greater risk due to psychological and social factors. Returning to hypertension as a major risk factor for CHF, another risk factor for hypertension is chronic psychological stress. Living in a community that is subject to continued racial discrimination in many areas of life is itself a source of great stress among blacks and explains their differential susceptibility to hypertension and therefore to CHF.[27]

6. Blacks and whites do not differ biologically, or in relation to access to medical care, insofar as CHF is concerned. But there are (physical) environmental factors that predispose toward developing CHF, such as living in areas that are subject to certain sorts of air and water pollution. Due to extensive *de facto* housing segregation in the United States, blacks are much more likely than whites to inhabit neighborhoods where these forms of pollution exist.[28]

This list is rendered more complex by its not being mutually exclusive; indeed it seems more likely than not that several if not all of these causal factors may be partly responsible for the disparities observed.

These possible causes have vastly different ethical, as well as policy implications. If #1 is true, then no one is currently to blame for the higher rate of CHF in blacks; it is as close as possible to being a brute fact of the natural world. If #4 is true, then the health-care system itself seems directly responsible for the disparity. If #3 is true, then many would argue that the black victims of CHF are themselves responsible.

Sorting out which factors, or combinations of factors, may be playing a causal role in the disparity would seem to be a matter for careful empirical investigation. How could bioethics assist? First, bioethicists could join forces with their empirical colleagues in warning against premature closure. Our society seems quite impatient to decide "the answer" to any given social problem, and too often has limited tolerance for answers that start out, "it depends" or "there are a number of interacting causes." Such tendencies increase the risk that we will get it wrong and propose ineffective policies. That in turn will further delay the day when the disparities are reduced or eliminated. On the other hand, it is also possible that we could encounter failure of closure. Some who have recently opposed measures to reverse global warming have hidden behind the rationalization that the science is still imprecise and imperfect, and that more studies are needed, even after prestigious scientific groups have pronounced that there is more than adequate evidence to view the situation as dire. Similar foot-dragging could occur around health disparities, if the necessary solutions indicated by the data turn out to be contrary to the interests of some powerful group.

Second, because the different causal explanations imply very different things for personal and institutional responsibility, the players in this drama do not start out equally receptive to all explanations—the "honest null hypothesis" that scientists love to talk about. It is only human to favor an answer that shows that somebody else is responsible for something bad happening. Also, to many physicians and medical scientists, Explanation #1 sounds much more legitimately "medical" than Explanation #5. Given the opportunity, these scientists will design experiments that systematically look for genetic answers and that exclude from view any potential psychosocial answers.[29]

What about the physicians' reluctance to accept an explanation that depicts them as engaging in practices that are somehow racially discriminatory? An instructive study suggests how hard such an explanation may be to tease out—how deeply below the surface such factors may be hidden. A psychological test, the Implicit Association Test, has been developed and widely validated. This test allows the detection of unconscious racial or other bias by requiring the test subject to register associations and likes/dislikes so rapidly that the conscious filters of behavior are bypassed. A person may say, quite honestly, that she does not like black people more than she likes white people. The test will then present her with pairs of photos showing white and black faces, asking her which person she likes better, and forcing her to make these choices at high speed. If the results show a highly statistically significant preference for black faces over white faces, the experimenter concludes that this subject has a racial bias that she is not consciously aware of.

The study presented a group of residents with the case of a 50-year-old man, "Mr. Thomas," who comes to the emergency room complaining of chest pain. The "right" answer to the case is that Mr. Thomas has a high likelihood of an acute coronary syndrome or heart attack and should under the circumstances receive a thrombolytic (clot-dissolving) drug immediately. The "Mr. Thomas" presented to half the residents was white; for the other half, the patient was black.

Similar to previous studies, the residents recommended the thrombolytic drug for "Mr. Thomas" less often when he has black than when he was white, even though they judged it equally likely in both cases that coronary syndrome was the correct diagnosis. The residents also denied any conscious bias against or dislike of black patients. When they took a modified version of the Implicit Association Test, however, a significant number of the residents showed an unconscious preference for whites over blacks. And the extent of that bias was directly correlated with how likely the resident was to recommend the drug for the white Mr. Thomas or to deny that drug to the black Mr. Thomas.[30]

It seems quite likely that these investigators have uncovered a possible cause for health disparities in a great many settings. What they discovered is something that the involved physicians are not consciously aware of and explicitly deny, in good faith. The careful and unusual methodology required to identify the hidden bias suggests just how deeply it was hidden. With no one being consciously aware of the bias, it is easy to see how numerous policy reforms, aimed at eliminating bias in treatment, might have no effect.

Bioethicists need to join in the effort to beware studies that purport to exclude a causal explanation—especially one that the group performing the study would prefer not to be true. If the methods used have not dug deeply enough, it may be premature to take that causal hypothesis off the table.[31]

*Policy implementation.* Once we know that disparities exist, and think that we understand their causes, we must design, implement, and evaluate new policies to correct them. At this stage, several ethical questions may emerge.

How are we to prioritize policies when resources are scarce and many different quality and safety initiatives are vying for attention? Depending on the causal mechanisms identified, part of the answer may lie in arguments about justice. Other things being equal, if an existing health-care practice causes or perpetuates injustice, that would seem to be an argument in favor of seeking to correct that practice before we might address other aspects of the health-care system needing improvement.

The fact that some health disparities may signal serious injustice does not mean that we should uncritically jump onto *any* health disparities bandwagon. Commercial interests have discovered the public-relations value of "health disparities" and have in some cases seduced well-meaning minority health advocates to their causes. BiDil, the first drug approved by the Food and Drug Administration for a single racial group (to treat CHF in African-Americans), provides an unfortunate example. The company first designed a clinical trial for purposes of its own commercial advantages rather than to answer the scientifically most important questions; then priced a drug which is basically the combination of two older generic drugs at four times the generic price; and finally tried to attack those who objected as being anti–minority health.[32]

Finally, some methods employed to try to reduce or eliminate disparities might raise their own ethical questions. For example, January Angeles and Stephen A. Somers (in a report previously cited) propose using pay-for-performance incentives to address health disparities. They correctly note that pay-for-performance plans are not without their own dangers. They therefore warn that any such incentive plan must be designed to watch carefully for unintended consequences. Perhaps the most obvious danger is that a health plan will get its disparity numbers to look better in the short run by allowing quality to deteriorate for majority patients. Thus, Angeles and Somers propose that any incentive to reduce disparities should be tried to other incentives that hinge on maintaining overall quality.[33]

## :: Conclusion

This chapter has surveyed only a few of the issues that might arise in health care around race and ethnicity. I have tied to show that the conceptual tools that the bioethicist brings to the table can address these issues in several helpful ways. Those conceptual tools are not the exclusive property of bioethics, so scholars in other disciplines could often address these matters in quite a satisfactory manner as well. Still, bioethics does have something to offer, and the number and complexity of the issues could keep the field fruitfully occupied for some time to come. In order to apply the tools to best advantage in the health disparities area, bioethicists would have to work very closely with scientists studying the empirical aspects of health disparities, and also with policymakers trying to design useful interventions.

1. I don't mean to deny that there is a group in bioethics that would dispute the position I have outlined, and that holds a more libertarian position on the so-called "right to health care" for a variety of reasons. See, for example, Engelhardt HT Jr. Rights to health care, social justice, and fairness in health care allocations: frustrations in the face of finitude. In: *The foundations of bioethics*, 2ⁿᵈ ed. New York: Oxford University Press, 1996, pp. 375–410.

2. Porter E. The divisions that tighten the purse strings. *New York Times*, April 29, 2007: Sect. 3, p. 4.

3. For a more detailed discussion of whether cultural relativism is a viable position in ethics, see Chapter 7.

4. Garcia JLA. Revisiting African American perspectives on biomedical ethics: distinctiveness and other questions. In: Prograis L Jr., Pellegrino ED, eds. *African American bioethics: culture, race, and identity*. Washington, DC: Georgetown University Press, 2007, pp. 1–23; list of characteristics, p. 4.

5. Garcia goes on to argue than this distinctively African-American bioethics would of necessity reject such practices as euthanasia, assisted suicide, abortion, and any destruction of human embryos, "as a logical and proper extension of our continuing struggles against racial violence and injustice"; Garcia JLA. Revisiting African American perspectives on biomedical ethics: distinctiveness and other questions, pp. 1–23, quote on p. 14. I fail to follow the logic of this particular set of conclusions.

6. Garcia JLA. Revisiting African American perspectives on biomedical ethics: distinctiveness and other questions, pp. 1–23, quote on p. 4.

7. For examples, see Schwartz RS. Racial profiling in medical research. *N Engl J Med* 344:1392–3, 2001 (denying value of racial categories in medical research); Burchard EG, Ziv E, Coyle N, et al. The importance of race and ethnic background in biomedical research and clinical practice. *N Engl J Med* 348:1170–75, 2003; Risch N, Burchard E, Ziv E, et al. Categorization of humans in biomedical research: genes, race and disease. *Genome Biol* 3(7):comment 2007 [epub], 2002 (defending medical utility of geographic race).

8. Jackson DZ. Another era of willful white ignorance. *Boston Globe*, July 4, 2007:A9.

9. One such effort was the Racial Privacy Initiative, California Ballot Measure #14, 2001–2 (which was unsuccessful).

10. Miller BL. Autonomy and the refusal of lifesaving treatment. *Hastings Cent Rep* 11(4):22–28, 1981.

11. I draw here on a paper co-authored with Linda M. Hunt and Clarence C. Gravlee, "Making Sense of Race," presented at the conference "Rethinking Inequalities and Differences in Medicine," Vanderbilt University, April 29–March 1, 2005.

12. I am grateful to Linda M. Hunt and Clarence C. Gravlee for this observation.

13. Hahn RA. Why race is differently classified on U.S. birth and infant death certificates: an examination of two hypotheses. *Epidemiol* 10:108–11,

1999; Jones CP. Invited commentary: "race," racism, and the practice of epidemiology. *Am J Epidemiol* 154:299–304, 2001.

14. See the section below on health disparities for a discussion of the ethical questions involved in gathering racially identified data for that purpose.

15. Analysis: a correspondent finds Afghans' optimism waning. *NPR Morning Edition*, June 28, 2007; http://www.npr.org/templates/story/story.php?storyId=11480909 (accessed June 28, 2007).

16. For an equally smug rejection of the value of "whiteness" for bioethics, see: Navel-gazing: bioethics and the unbearable whiteness of being [editorial]. *New Atlantis*, No. 2, Summer 2003:98–100.

17. Pitts L. Replying to those e-mails about Vick. *Miami Herald*, August 12, 2007, http://www.miamiherald.com/living/columnists/leonard_pitts/story/199338.html (accessed August 24, 2007).

18. Myser C. Differences from somewhere: the normativity of whiteness in bioethics in the United States. *Am J Bioeth* 2003; 3(2):1–11; quoting Baldwin J. On being white...and other lies. In: Roediger DR, ed. *Black on white: black writers on what it means to be white*. New York: Schocken Books, 1984.

19. Todd KH, Samaroo N, Hoffman JR. Ethnicity as a risk factor for inadequate emergency department analgesia. *JAMA* 269:1537–39, 1993. A later study in Atlanta showed a similar disparity in pain management between white and black patients with long-bone fractures; Todd KH, Deaton C, D'Adamo AP, et al.. Ethnicity and analgesic practice. *Ann Emerg Med* 35: 11–16, 2000.

20. The most extensive and influential review of health disparities is: Institute of Medicine. *Unequal treatment: confronting racial and ethnic disparities in health care*. Washington, DC: National Academies Press, 2003.

21. Given the importance of the "medical home" concept as discussed in Chapter 3, it is of interest that some evidence suggests that providing minority patients with a medical home is effective in reducing health disparities; Beal AC, Doty MM, Hernandez SE, et al. *Closing the divide: how medical homes promote equity in health care: results from the Commonwealth Fund 2006 health care quality survey*. Vol. 62 (June 27, 2007); http://www.commonwealthfund.org/publications/publications_show.htm?doc_id=506814& (accessed August 25, 2007).

22. Daniels N. Equity and population health: toward a broader bioethics agenda. *Hastings Cent Rep* 36(4):22–35, 2006.

23. Daniels N. Equity and population health: toward a broader bioethics agenda; see especially pp. 23–26.

24. Angeles J, Somers SA. From policy to action: addressing racial and ethnic disparities at the ground-level. *Center for Health Care Strategies Issue Brief*, August 2007, http://www.chcs.org/usr_doc/From_Policy_to_Action.pdf (accessed August 25, 2007); quote on p. 3.

25. Angeles J, Somers SA. From policy to action: addressing racial and ethnic disparities at the ground-level; quote on p. 3.

26. King P. Race, equity, health policy, and the African American community. In: Prograis L Jr., Pellegrino ED, eds. *African American bioethics: culture,*

*race, and identity.* Washington, DC: Georgetown University Press, 2007:67–92.

27. I place "biological" in scare quotes here because we must assume that these psychosocial factors must have biological consequences if they result in a disease such as CHF. Chronic stress has been shown to change the secretion of corticosteroid hormones from the adrenal gland, and these hormones can affect cardiovascular function and blood pressure.

28. This factor is mentioned only in passing by Normal Daniels: Daniels N. Equity and population health: toward a broader bioethics agenda. *Hastings Cent Rep* 36(4):22–35, 2006.

29. Sankar P. Cho MK, Condit CM, et al. Genetic research and health disparities. *JAMA* 291:2985–89, 2004.

30. Green AR, Carney DR, Pallin DJ, et al. Implicit bias among physicians and its prediction of thrombolysis decisions for black and white patients. *J Gen Intern Med* 22:1231–8, 2007. One possible objection to this study is that the methodology was *too* subtle, and detected a bias that was buried so deep that it could not possibly affect the actual behavior of the subjects. The reply to this objection is the findings of the study itself—that the bias *did* affect actual behavior, as it predicted to a very high level of statistical significance the withholding of the preferred treatment from the black patient.

31. Another example of this premature closure, from the experience with BiDil (to be discussed later in this chapter), is well addressed by Jonathan Kahn. Some of the scientists who wished to defend genetic factors in blacks as an explanation for their excess rate of CHF claimed that they had carefully looked for psychosocial explanatory factors and had found none. In fact they had looked only at a handful of variables and had done nothing resembling an exhaustive search for psychosocial causes: Kahn J. How a drug becomes "ethnic": law, commerce, and the production of racial categories in medicine. *Yale J Health Policy Law Ethics* 4:1–46, 2004.

32. On the BiDil story, see Kahn J. How a drug becomes "ethnic": law, commerce, and the production of racial categories in medicine; Brody H, Hunt LM. BiDil: assessing a race-based pharmaceutical. *Ann Fam Med* 4:556–60, 2006; Bibbins-Domingo K, Fernandez A. BiDil for heart failure in black patients: implications of the U.S. Food and Drug Administration approval. *Ann Intern Med* 146:52–6, 2007. The company's marketing efforts so far appear largely to have failed, and many insurance plans are refusing to cover this expensive drug. Sadly, this seems to mean that many black patients who might benefit from this drug combination are not today receiving it. See also Delancey DB. AIDSVAX and clinical trials: HIV/AIDS vaccine research and the Tuskegee Syphilis Study. In: Quirke V, Slinn J (eds.) *Twentieth-century perspectives on pharmaceuticals.* Oxford: Peter Lang, 2008.

33. Angeles J, Somers SA. From policy to action: addressing racial and ethnic disparities at the ground-level. *Center for Health Care Strategies Issue Brief,* August 2007, http://www.chcs.org/usr_doc/From_Policy_to_Action.pdf (accessed August 25, 2007). See Chapter 4 for more on the ethical issues raised by pay-for-performance (P4P) schemes.

# 9 ⠿
# Disabilities

In October, 2004, I was moved to offer an apology. When the case of David Rivlin was heard by a Michigan court in the 1980s, I had thought of it at the time as a typical "right to refuse life-sustaining treatment" case, such that all right-thinking individuals would support the principle of respect for patient autonomy. After I had become better sensitized to some of the concerns raised by advocates for persons with disabilities, I regretted my initial reaction. It now seemed more plausible to me that Rivlin might have wished to remain alive, even with quadriplegia and ventilator-dependent, if only he could have received better and more humane services that would have given him some meaningful options for living his life.

I expressed my apology in what I would have thought was about the most obscure venue that I might have chosen—a weekly alternative newspaper, the *Lansing City Pulse,* in which an occasional health-related column of mine appeared.[1] I was not at all ready for the reaction. I promptly began to receive e-mails from around the country. It seems that that column was immediately picked up and circulated by several websites, and eventually publications, devoted to disabilities-related issues. Apparently, for that audience, the idea that a bioethicist would apologize for getting something wrong with regard to a disabilities issue was major news.

I mention this personal anecdote simply to illustrate one point— how the relationship between the bioethics and the disabilities communities has become severely strained. The date at which the strain developed can probably be pinpointed—the Bloomington, Indiana,

Baby Doe case of 1982. Bioethicists tended to support, in that situation, the rights of parents of an infant with Down syndrome and esophageal atresia to refuse surgery and to allow the infant to die—though, relatively soon after, the President's Commission took the position that Down syndrome was an insufficiently serious birth defect to warrant a decision to refuse life-prolonging surgery.[2] Disabilities advocates were shocked that a group that considered themselves spokespersons for *ethics* in medicine would favor such blatant discrimination against an infant with a disability. As I will describe below, there has been little love lost between those two camps since.

My goals in this chapter are, first, to suggest the relevance of the feminist model of power disparities to the disabilities setting; and second, to suggest that bioethics has a lot to gain by re-opening useful dialogue with students of disabilities. I will start by reviewing the social conception of disabilities. I will then discuss a theory of justice that seems particularly promising (as well as expansive) for addressing persons with disabilities. Finally I will return to two areas of tension between bioethics and disabilities advocates to see in what practical directions a re-opened dialogue might take us.

## ∷ A Thought Experiment

Imagine that you are a person of normal eyesight. Tomorrow morning you awaken to find that the world has undergone a substantial change. Everything that used to be written in the standard alphabet is now in Braille. The newspaper delivered to your doorstep in the morning is in Braille. So are all the street signs and billboards that you pass on your trip to work. When you get to work, you discover that your computer monitor has been replaced by a tactile Braille board. All the documents in your office are in Braille.

It seems likely that at least two things will happen as a result of this overnight transformation. First, your ability to function in the world will be markedly reduced. The are many things that you could do with ease yesterday, that today you will be unable to do at all, or can do only with extreme difficulty. Probably you will feel that there is something *unfair* in all this. After all, it is not as if you suddenly became stupid, or lost all your innate talents, or forgot all of your education, or became grossly uncoordinated. It seems quite clear that it is nothing about *you* that has suddenly robbed you of your ability to function at an adequate level.

Second, quite apart from the ability to function at any given level in the world, you are probably going to feel ill-treated, perhaps even violated, by these new arrangements of the world. You know from your own past experience that there is nothing *natural* about the standard alphabet being in near-universal use on one day, and Braille suddenly replacing it the next day. These are differences in social arrangements, and somebody, somewhere, must have chosen to make this alteration. You have been rendered seriously non-functional, not by some fate of nature, but as a result of social choice. It is quite natural that you should deeply resent whoever made that choice.

Your sense of being treated unfairly and of being ill-used is not mitigated as you overhear some remarks among blind people. "Those non-Braille readers are whining again, I hear. *We* had to learn how to read Braille many years ago. You didn't hear us griping about it. For us to get ahead in the world, we had to take responsibility for ourselves and work hard. *Those* people seem to think they should have special privileges handed to them, just because they are different and because they complain louder than anyone else."

There is nothing novel about this thought experiment. It is no different than the learning exercises commonly designed by disabilities advocates to educate the rest of us about what daily life is like for a person with a disability, by getting us to remain in a wheelchair, or to try to see through some special goggles, for a period of time. It is the old adage about walking a mile in the other person's moccasins. I employ it here to illustrate a concept that most people at first find counter-intuitive—the social model of disability.[3] Our usual way of thinking about the problems faced by a person with a disability—a wheelchair user with a spinal cord injury, for example—is that it is her physical state that is the root cause of whatever her functional problems may be. "Fixing" her disability would require something that would regenerate the nerves in her spinal cord. Her inability to function is certainly not due to anything we have done, or any choices we have made.

The social model objects that many persons with disabilities could function quite well, compared to how they are able to function today, if the world were designed differently, and various barriers to their functioning were removed. The fact that the world is designed in the way that it is, and the fact that these barriers exist, reflects a series of social choices and actions. There is nothing in nature that says that streets should not have curb cuts, that buildings should not have ramps or elevators, or that city buses should not have wheelchair lifts. And if we "normal" people were on the receiving end for a change—if we suddenly found the world designed to favor people who were *differently abled* from ourselves (as in the thought experiment)—we would instantly perceive this to be true.

The thought experiment is designed to confront us with the question: since we can as easily imagine a world in which everything is written in Braille, as a world like the one we live in today, according to what ethical principle could we say that the world *should* be as it is?[4] The only vaguely plausible ethical principle that I could imagine being brought forth, is one that relies on the fact that "normally" sighted people are statistically much more common than blind people. But I would imagine that no one would find satisfactory an "ethical principle" that said that the way we ought to treat people depends on whether they are in a numerical majority or minority.

The thought experiment further shows why the commonly heard objection, "Of course it would be *nice* to offer accommodations to various sorts of persons with disabilities, but we simply cannot afford the cost," is question-begging. Certain things are simply the cost of doing business in the world, and are widely understood to be so, as long as it is "normally" abled people for whom the social world is designed. We could, for instance, no doubt save a lot of money if all highways were paved with gravel and we chose to drive down these roads at 15 miles an hour. No one seems to object to the costs of insisting on concrete roads that allow us to travel at 70 miles per hour.

The importance of the social dimension is further demonstrated by a distinction among *impairment, disability,* and *handicap.* Most medical conditions that are usually thought of as "disabilities" can be dealt with in this framework. By way of example, consider a patient undergoing post-stroke rehabilitation. The stroke has caused significant weakness on one side of the body (hemiparesis). This condition represents an *impairment,* a dysfunction of a part of the body. As a result of the impairment, the person might have *disabilities.* He cannot, for instance, walk without using an assist device, or do many things with one hand that he used to be able to do. The response of the society round him will then determine whether he also has a *handicap.* A handicap would occur if, for instance, he was previously employed, but cannot now return to work.

The importance of these distinctions is shown by research on quality of life as perceived by persons with disabilities. Medical people generally assume that the more severe one's impairment or disability, the worse the quality of life that will be experienced. This turns out generally to be untrue. Instead, one's quality of life is almost completely bound up with handicap. The extent to which society will or will not make accommodations, the degree to which one's disabilities do or do not prevent social functioning and integration, determine the quality of life.[5]

According to the social model of disability, which appears to me to be plausible for a good number of (but not all) cases, certain bad outcomes in terms of an individual's ability to function in accordance with his level of talent and education are the result of social choices. According to the common-sense view of disability, those same bad outcomes are dictated by the physical nature of the person's impairment. When we systematically confuse social choices with "facts of nature," it would seem to be a fairly standard move for philosophical ethics to point out this flaw in reasoning and seek to correct it. If bioethics has not raised its voice louder to call attention to this problem in thinking about disabilities, this might well suggest to disabilities advocates that bioethicists are not much interested in their concerns.

## ✷ Justice and Persons with Disabilities

What theoretical underpinnings might best support a robust concern for the well-being of persons with disabilities? Martha Nussbaum has offered a promising framework.[6]

Nussbaum views her enterprise as extending the theory of justice provided by John Rawls, which she views as the most developed theory in the liberal social-contract tradition. She believes that Rawls's theory is especially powerful because of its grounding in Kantian ethics as well as in social-contract theory. The Kantian element helps to assure that the dignity of the individual can never be compromised in the name of some general social good.

For all of its strengths, Rawls's theory of justice can never be a satisfactory theory of why we owe full respect and citizenship to persons with disabilities. The theory's defects arise both from its Kantian and its social-contract elements. On the Kantian side, human dignity is equated with the capability to make rational choices. This implies that anyone with severe mental disabilities, in particular, can never be worthy of full respect. On the social-contract side, Rawls follows his predecessors since Locke in insisting that a theory of justice requires that a group of free, equal, and independent contractors agree to it as securing a level of mutual advantage that they could not achieve otherwise. But this condition is implausible when applied to those with serious disabilities. Some could be helped by the appropriate services to become fully functioning members of society, with a degree of economic productivity that could pay back the society for the services extended. But those with more severe disabilities could never realistically be expected to "pay back" in this economic sense. Contractors conceived of as equal and independent (that is, *not* subject to serious disabilities) could never find it to their *personal* advantage to provide the needed level of care.

As Nussbaum notes, Rawls admits all these difficulties with his theory when it comes to dealing with citizens who lack the "normal" range of physical and mental abilities. He treats this as a problem that cannot be dealt with at the level of determining the basic structure of society, which is where his contracting occurs (in the hypothetical Original Position). Once the basic structure of society has been determined, these problems, Rawls thinks, can be dealt with satisfactorily at the later, legislative stage.[7] Nussbaum argues that this so-called solution is inadequate. A social-contract theory of justice imagines parties freely agreeing to a basic structure for society which they then further agree to be bound by and to live under. They choose a structure *by* themselves and *for* themselves. By saying to persons with disabilities, "We will exclude you from the social contract arrangements, but will get around to your needs later on," we declare them to be neither the sorts of persons who choose the structure of society, nor the sorts of persons for whom it is chosen. If our goal is their fullest possible participation and flourishing in the society that results, we have hardly made a promising start.

As a corrective extension to Rawls's liberal theory, Nussbaum proposes a theory of justice focused on a list of "central human capabilities":[8]

- A reasonable life span
- Bodily health
- Bodily integrity and safety
- Being able to use one's senses, to imagine, think, and reason
- Being able to experience the range of human emotions
- Practical reasoning, the ability to plan one's life
- Engaging in social affiliations and interactions

- Living in the world of nature in fellowship with other plant and animal species
- Opportunities to play and to enjoy leisure
- Reasonable control over one's political and material environment, including rights to political participation

What makes a life a fully human life, in accord with human dignity, is the opportunity to exercise all (or at least most) of these capabilities. Bare Kantian rationality turns out to be an incomplete account of human capabilities. A just society, on this theory, will seek to provide to each person the opportunity to achieve a reasonable minimum of the functioning of each separate capacity. The different capacities are incommensurable; a society cannot, for instance, strip persons of basic political rights and make up for it by giving them better-quality health care.

Nussbaum's corrective to Rawls's Kantian element is to insist that we attend to the deeper and more important idea of the dignity of each human being, rather than to the more limited idea of autonomous, rational choice. Her corrective to the social-contract element in Rawls is to keep hold of the idea of freely choosing a basic structure of society, without insisting that the contractors be equal and independent, and that they agree to a structure solely out of a concern for their mutual advantage. Nussbaum reminds us that an exclusive concern with "independent" contractors valorizes one part of the "normal" human life span to the detriment of other portions:

> Thus, in the design of the political conception of the person, out of which basic political principles grow, we build in an acknowledgment that we are needy temporal animal beings who begin as babies and end, often, in other forms of dependency. We draw attention to these areas of vulnerability, insisting that rationality and sociability are themselves temporal, having growth, maturity, and (if time permits) decline. We acknowledge, as well, that the kind of sociability that is fully human includes symmetrical relations, such as those that are central for Rawls, but also relations of more or less extreme asymmetry; we insist that the nonsymmetrical relations can still contain reciprocity and truly human functioning.[9]

Nussbaum suggests that when we choose a basic structure of society that leaves no room for persons with disabilities, we also effectively exclude a large and humanly important chunk of the life span of the "normal" person, which is equally marked by dependency, asymmetrical relations, and a need for care: "And bodily need, including the need for care, is a feature of our rationality and our sociability; it is one aspect of our dignity, then, rather than something to be contrasted with it."[10]

What about individuals who are so severely impaired that some or even all of the capabilities on the list seem out of reach? Nussbaum admits that, "if the entirety of a group of major human capabilities is irrevocably and entirely cut off," the result is "sufficiently significant to constitute the death of anything like a characteristic human form of life."[11] This is applicable, she says, to (former) persons in a persistent vegetative state, and to anencephalic infants. Thus Nussbaum sides with the majority of bioethicists against some of the more extreme disabilities advocates, who would argue that stopping the feeding tube of a patient in persistent vegetative state is an example of intolerable discrimination against persons with disabilities. Once we move beyond such extreme cases, however, the proper role of the just society is to do what can be done to develop and nurture those capabilities that exist, at least up to a minimum level of support.

To draw out the implications of a capabilities approach, let us consider in more detail the last capability on the list, which includes rights to political participation. This would include the right to vote. It seems possible at the outset to divide persons with disabilities into three broad categories—those who clearly possess the intellectual capabilities we normally associate with the ability to choose among political candidates; those who clearly lack those intellectual capabilities, and would continue to lack them despite any intervention we could design; and those in a middle group where the answer may be unclear.

We would seem to have obvious duties toward people in the first group, to assure that those with the intellectual capacity to cast a vote are not impeded by any physical or sensory barriers. Polling places must be easily accessible to all who wish to use them, and absentee ballots easily obtainable for those who do not. Citizens with sight limitations should have useable ballots available to them.

Those in the middle or questionable-ability group should be the subject of some inquiry and investigation. Are there any long-term changes in the way these people are offered educational services, for example, that might make a difference in whether they later achieve a clear intellectual ability to participate in voting? If so, then we discern an obligation to alter the educational system to make this possible. The point is that we have identified a way in which this group of individuals could be enabled to function, so as to support a fully human life with dignity. That creates an expectation of justice that entails a strong (though rebuttable) duty to provide the needed resources, at least up to an agreed-upon threshold level. In a society as wealthy as ours, it would be hard to rebut such a duty simply on grounds of cost—especially since so many other nations enjoying a similar or even lower level of wealth appear to do much more than we do at present.

That would, finally, seem to exclude only those who clearly and permanently lack the intellectual ability to choose among candidates and cast a vote meaningfully. Are we done with that group? Nussbaum would argue that we still need to explore the possibility of creating a system where others acting as proxies might exercise at least a partial right to vote on their behalf. She would be strongly opposed to appointing a guardian to do things that the person herself might do on her own, given the appropriate resources and assistance. But in other cases she would propose that the guardian be allowed to exercise limited rights on behalf of the person with disabilities, rather than have those rights simply disappear. She alludes to policies recently enacted in Israel, Sweden, and Germany as models that we might consider emulating.[12]

Nussbaum cites examples from other nations of innovative programs to better address the capabilities of persons with various disabilities, and also the needs of those who provide care for them. She even endorses the German precedent, of requiring national service from all youth—either two years of military service or three years of alternative service, much of which is care work for vulnerable citizens. It is not only that inducting young people to the work of caring for persons with disabilities allows society to get the work done by a relatively energetic and cheap labor force. Nussbaum believes that there are real advantages to introducing to both genders the notion of the value and dignity of caregiving at that age—"this experience could be expected to shape their attitudes in political debates and in family life."[13]

One could object here that Nussbaum's proposal seems far too sweeping, so that the resources to be diverted to the care of persons with disabilities sound limitless. An alternative proposal would hold that it is simply unrealistic to try to apply the complete list of ten basic capabilities to persons with severe mental impairment. We need, instead, what one might call a "long capabilities list" for the rest of us, and a "short capabilities list" for those with severe disabilities. Nussbaum explicitly rejects this two-tier proposal. First, there is the slippery slope problem. In the past, whenever a two-tier approach has been recommended, it has proved all too easy to conclude that since those with the more severe disabilities could not possibly benefit from some proposed services, these same services would be equally useless for many with less severe disabilities. Ironically, Nussbaum argues, insisting on a single "long list" for everyone demands that each be treated as an individual, and not stereotyped as a member of a class. Since the long list describes the basic necessities of a life with dignity *for everyone,* we must carefully go down the list *for each individual,* to decide very carefully what capabilities do and do not apply given the severity of that individual's disabilities.[14]

Nussbaum adds that there is a deeper reason, apart from the slippery slope, to insist on the "long list" for all. It is very easy to fall back into our notions of what is statistically "normal," and to assume that it is a brute biological fact that persons with severe disabilities lack some of the basic human capabilities. By contrast, if we took the "long list" view seriously, Nussbaum argues that we would regard these lacks as *unfortunate* from a perspective of justice. This account of justice reminds us that persons with serious disabilities are *people like us,* and not a different species of animal. It forces us to realize that what separates the rest of us from these people is not a wide gulf, but a series of infinitely subtle gradations.[15]

Nussbaum's theory of justice is bioethics-friendly in the way that it adopts multiple, relatively concrete outcomes as the indices of social justice. How just any society is at any given time is determined by how well it provides for a multiplicity of human capabilities. This determination in turn requires that we examine both what is actually possible, given the nature and limits posed by specific disabilities; and also which, among many possible interventions and services, actually activates the capabilities in question to the greatest degree and with the greatest efficiency in the use of scarce social resources. Nussbaum also warns us against too great a devotion to the ethic of care. We ought not shower a person with disabilities with care when we could have been making her independent and no longer in need of care of that sort. All these sorts of practical determinations seem to be of the sort that bioethicists have been used to grappling with in various health-care settings. We cannot presume to speak on behalf of persons with disabilities, but we can facilitate the needed dialogue.


## ∷ How Might Bioethics Change?

What would the practical world of bioethics look like, if we took to heart the concerns of advocates for persons with disabilities, and newer theoretical work such as Nussbaum's? How, that is, might we best translate

Nussbaum's insights from theory to practice? There are two areas where bioethics activity has especially come under fire from the disabilities community—end-of-life care and resource allocation. Other areas could be listed as well, but the two major areas are sufficient for illustration here.[16]

*End-of-life care.* Adrienne Asch has offered a moderate, thoughtful set of suggestions as to how bioethics might improve the way we address end-of-life care issues. Contrary to the fears of some bioethicists, and distancing herself from the strident rhetoric of groups like Not Dead Yet, Asch argues that adopting a disabilities perspective does not entail accepting a sanctity-of-life view or jumping into bed politically with religious fundamentalists. Indeed, the primary reforms that Asch calls for appear quite modest.[17] First, bioethicists should be active among health professionals in reversing the stereotype that any physical or mental impairment automatically leads to a lessened quality of life and diminished human dignity. Included in this shift in awareness is the realization that the ambivalence of the temporarily-able-bodied toward the person with disabilities can easily lead to an unconscious desire to resolve our own discomfort by seeking the other's elimination.

This does not mean that a wish to forgo life-sustaining treatment by a person with a disability should never be honored. It does mean that the threshold for acceptance of the basic autonomy of the individual's choice needs to be recalibrated. All bioethicists would look askance at a classic case once proposed by Bruce Miller, in which a young man, previously in excellent health, is discovered in an emergency room to have a bacterial meningitis probably completely curable with intravenous antibiotics; yet the patient refuses all treatment and indicates that he wishes instead to die.[18] Most of us would set the bar very high in that case, before we would agree that the patient's expressed wish is *truly* autonomous and so demands our acquiescence. By contrast, if a ninety-year-old patient with a terminal illness refuses a painful treatment that might extend her life by a few days, we would have a correspondingly low threshold for declaring her capable of an autonomous decision. Asch's request is that we adjust the bar higher when dealing with cases of persons with disabilities, and set the bar especially high when the length of life still possible is long—as was true, for example, in the widely publicized case of Elizabeth Bouvia.[19]

What, exactly, does "setting the bar higher" mean? Asch's recommendation is that an apparently rational person who registers a desire to refuse life-prolonging therapy due to a disability, despite the possibility of prolonged survival, needs at least two interventions. First, those knowledgeable about disabilities services should review the case to assure that all appropriate resources had been considered. An example is provided by the case of David Rivlin, which prompted the apology I described at the beginning of the chapter. Rivlin, 38 years old and quadriplegic, was allowed by the court to die by disconnecting his ventilator. One of the main reasons he wished to die was his hopelessness at facing a life that consisted of staring at the four walls of his nursing-home room. Few noted that there was no reason he should have been confined in that way, and that at the time the case was reviewed, there were services available to allow him to move into his own apartment and to travel to some extent with a portable ventilator. In hindsight, the case was mismanaged by both the physicians and the court, by not taking those alternatives for improving Rivlin's quality of life much more seriously.

Second, a person with a similar disability, who has managed to survive with the help of the life-prolonging treatment in question, should be sought to visit with the patient and to make sure that the patient has an accurate view of what life might be like in such a situation. Finally, and consistent with both of the previous interventions, hospital ethics committees and similar groups should make more of an effort to assure that persons with a deep understanding of disabilities issues are among their members.

*Resource allocation.* The sorts of cases that have given disabilities advocates the chills about bioethicists's end-of-life pontifications illustrate the concerns those advocates express about the ethics of resource allocation. Bioethics seems ready to declare that persons with disabilities uniformly suffer a poor quality of life, and therefore if one of them asks for a type of treatment that would result in an early death, respect for their autonomy requires that this wish speedily be granted—without wasting time by inquiring too deeply whether the choice is truly an informed, rational one and whether all alternatives have adequately been explored. It makes perfect sense that the same field of bioethics, faced with the problem of distributing limited health-care resources, would want those resources to go where they would produce the most benefit—and by definition, that could not include persons with disabilities, whose quality of life is so low that prolonging such a life can hardly be doing them any favors. Therefore, any time a bioethicist proposes a scheme for rationing limited health-care resources, a disabilities advocate stands ready to brand that scheme as a dastardly plot to eliminate persons with disabilities.[20]

On the face of it, the disabilities advocates would seem to have some cause for their alarm, quite apart from the poor performance of the bioethics crowd with regard to "right to die" cases such as Bouvia and Rivlin. For example, Norman Daniels and others writing on justice and resource allocation have identified a category of patient that presents special problems. These patients are described as being so severely afflicted that no matter how much health care is provided for them, at no matter how great an expense, their eventual level of function can never even begin to approach "normal" range—the criterion that Daniels favors as giving rise to a justice-based argument in support of an entitlement to health care.[21] Daniels and others have termed such patients "bottomless pits," capable of consuming resources to an infinite degree with no resultant benefit. Given that many of these "bottomless pits" would presumably be persons with severe disabilities, one can see how the use of such a term is hardly reassuring to disabilities advocates.

Can anything be done to bridge this conceptual divide? I believe that productive dialogue could begin, but it would require a fresh departure on both sides. I have already indicated ways in which bioethics needs to reform its views of persons with disabilities and of their "quality of life." Let me now suggest what has to happen on the disabilities side.

To my knowledge, no one on the disabilities end of this debate has attempted to do a cost estimate of what resources might be required to meet the legitimate needs of today's population of persons with disabilities in the United States. I here assume that persons with disabilities have health-care needs like everyone else and that a reasonable health-care system would provide funds sufficient to meet those needs, for hospitalizations, medicines, and so forth. Those resource needs are not what I am here referring to. Rather I assume that there is another set of needs that relate to the possible use of assistance technology, or assistance staff, to allow a person with a disability to function at a more satisfactory level—in Nussbaum's terms, to fulfill one or more of the basic human capabilities. Let us call this entire class of expenses "assistance costs." There is obviously going to be a gray zone between basic medical costs and assistance costs, but I do not believe that the gray area negates the basic conceptual point I wish to make.

If assistance costs were fully covered by our society, many good things would happen for persons with disabilities as well as for the rest of us. Many more such persons could find productive employment, living happier lives but also being economically more productive and so paying back in taxes some of the costs of both medical care and assistance. As more persons with disabilities functioned at a higher level, *and were seen by the rest of us to be functioning that way,* the social stigma attached to disability would be mitigated. The rest of us would be much less prone to equate having a disability with living a life of low quality. We would be much slower to jump to the conclusion that if such a person were seriously ill, the only humane thing to do would be to allow the person to die quickly. We would be much less prone to conclude that resources devoted to these patients were wasted, whether in the medical-care or in the assistance category. So on the face of it there are very strong considerations of both justice and prudence in favor of our society's paying those assistance costs as well as the basic medical costs.

Suppose now that we added up what those assistance costs are likely to be. In the crudest possible rendition, there are two possibilities. One is that the costs would turn out to be surprisingly low. This would be good news all around. It would be a very strong argument in favor of the absolute social priority of moving to allocate these funds as soon as possible. It would have been shown that, not only would spending this money have all the advantages we have reviewed above; but in addition, that the total sum needed is much less than most had feared. This would immediately remove the major objection to finding this sum of money and allocating it in this way.

The other possibility is that the total cost would be quite high. I suspect that this is actually not likely to be the case, as many countries (especially in Northern Europe) appear to spend considerably more than we do for disabilities assistance, and yet have come nowhere close to bankruptcy over it. But it is still possible that when we look hard at very expensive technologies such as computer-dependent assist devices, we will find a great deal that could significantly benefit a number of individuals with disabilities, but at a very high cost.

If this second scenario is the one that plays out, we still have strong arguments based on justice that we should somehow find this sum and allocate it for assistance purposes. But we would realize that the sum is truly immense and that there are serious practical barriers. It would be much more plausible in this scenario to argue that other matters of justice ought to take priority and so that the social fund for assistance could grow by only a modest amount per year, taking many years before it is fully funded.

Now, it is a large step from estimating the likely cost of this "assistance fund" to actually creating an entitlement program for persons with disabilities that was funded at that level. Many practical as well as conceptual problems would have to be addressed before we could get to that latter stage. So what is the point of calling for this cost estimate?

The main point that I wish to bring forward is that advocates for persons with disabilities, assuming that they accepted my challenge and made a good-faith effort to estimate the costs of the ideal assistance program, would have thereby agreed with the bioethics community that the correct way to think about the problem of resource allocation is to begin with the assumption of a finite resource pool. Let us imagine that our initial cost estimate was as generous as any advocate could ask for, and that just for good measure, we added a further 20 percent on top of that to cover unforeseen contingencies.[22] It would nevertheless be true that sooner or later, there would come a dispute about the allocation of resources *within* this assistance fund. Some advocates for persons with serious disabilities would claim that more of the funds should provide a certain sort of assistance for those individuals. Other advocates would see much greater benefits for persons with disabilities *overall* if the funds were spent on other things. According to these other advocates, the degree of benefit that would be enjoyed by the persons who would receive that expensive form of assistance is too small to justify the high cost. In short, these advocates would have, among themselves, the same sort of debate that we imagine non-disabled persons having about the allocation of health-care resources, if we had a transparent system of deliberation for resolving such issues in the health-care arena.

So long as they have not yet engaged in this cost-estimate exercise, which entails in turn the acceptance of the assumption of finite resources, disabilities advocates can have it both ways with the resource-allocation issue. On one hand, they can tell anecdotes about how cheap some forms of assistance are, and how our society ends up paying much higher costs as a result of refusing to provide those services than it would if the services were paid for. On the other hand, they can evade taking any hard stances on the need to allocate resources within the assistance pool, suggesting to their own constituency that ideally, everyone could have everything he or she wanted, and that there would be no limits of any sort, if only we could eliminate unjust discrimination against persons with disabilities. I believe it is the slippery, inconsistent nature of this position that leads bioethicists to conclude that they cannot have a useful dialogue with disabilities advocates over resource allocation.

And that, in turn, is what has led me to suggest that the cost-estimate exercise would help to clear the air and establish the dialogue that is needed.

There is, of course, one other move available to disabilities advocates. They could argue that my call for the cost estimate, and for the hypothetical "assistance fund," was itself based on assumptions that are unjust toward persons with disabilities. They would then feel justified in refusing to play my game.[23] But if this is their argument, they must give an account of themselves. Just what are those hidden assumptions, and in exactly what way are they unjust? The dialogue that could follow from those explanations might be as useful as anything that would follow from laying a cost estimate out on the table. So that route provides an alternative way that disabilities advocates could productively enter into dialogue with bioethicists. Either approach would be better than the current impasse, in which disabilities advocates suspect bioethicists of simply wishing to eliminate persons with disabilities in order to save money, and bioethicists suspect advocates of refusing to recognize the basic reality that health-care resources are not infinite.

End-of-life care and resource allocation are only two of a number of areas in bioethics where dialogue with advocates for persons with disabilities, and scholars in disabilities studies, might prove enlightening. I hold out no hope that this point that the two groups will ever see completely eye to eye on any of these issues. I do, however, look forward to being further educated as a result of the exchanges that are likely to occur.

NOTES TO CHAPTER 9

1. Brody H. A bioethicist offers an apology. *Lansing City Pulse*, October 6, 2004, http://www.lansingcitypulse.com/041006/features/health.asp (Accessed December 29, 2007).
2. U.S. President's Commission for the Study of Ethical Problems in Medicine and Biomedical and Behavioral Research. *Deciding to forego life-sustaining treatment*. Washington, DC: U.S. Government Printing Office, 1983.
3. Daniel Goldberg has provided a succinct summary of the social model of disability, along with a set of key references, on his Medical Humanities blog: http://www.medhumanities.org/2006/11/social_model_of.html (accessed September 8, 2008).
4. Today, in many places in the United States, progress has been made toward making the environment friendlier to the blind, utilizing a number of different sound and touch devices. Perhaps what I have in mind would be clearer if we were to ask for an ethical justification of our

social environment as it existed 10 to 15 years ago. On the other hand, I do not wish to suggest that the job is finished by any means.

5. Kothari S. Clinical (mis)judgments of quality of life after disability. *J Clin Ethics* 15:300–7, 2004. Kothari uses the distinctions among impairment, disability, and handicap suggested by the World Health Organization manual of classification (1980). He notes that WHO updated this manual and slightly revised these categories in 2001, but much of the existing research uses the 1980 categories.

6. Nussbaum MC. *Frontiers of justice: disability, nationality, species membership*. Cambridge, MA: Belknap-Harvard University Press, 2006, pp. 9–223.

7. Rawls J. *A theory of justice*. Cambridge, MA: Belknap-Harvard University Press, 1971; Rawls J. *Political liberalism*. New York: Columbia University Press, 1993.

8. Nussbaum MC. *Frontiers of justice: disability, nationality, species membership*, pp. 76–8. Nussbaum draws her approach to capabilities largely from the work of Amartya Sen.

9. Nussbaum MC. *Frontiers of justice: disability, nationality, species membership*, p. 160.

10. Nussbaum MC. *Frontiers of justice: disability, nationality, species membership*, p. 160. The radical nature of this statement deserves to be underlined, especially in contrast with a great deal of the early bioethics literature on the notion of "death with dignity." It was simply taken for granted in much of that literature that aging led to increased dependency on others, which automatically equaled a loss of dignity, which then generated a rational desire to die. The logical implication—that if dependency in aging equals a lack of basic human dignity, then infants and children should also be viewed as lacking human dignity—was seldom explored. The capabilities approach that Nussbaum favors could generate its own "dignified death" criteria, as it seems reasonable to conclude that in the natural unfolding of a human life, there will come a time when loss of capabilities is all that the future holds; but Nussbaum does not develop these implications.

11. Nussbaum MC. *Frontiers of justice: disability, nationality, species membership*, p. 181.

12. Nussbaum MC. Frontiers of justice: disability, nationality, species membership, pp. 195–9. Here, of course, one would have to tread warily. It is one thing to try to discover a method by which the civic interests of a person with disabilities can be exercised by a proxy; and quite another merely to announce that if you are the guardian for a person with a disability, you get to vote twice. The latter seems clearly unacceptable in a constitutional democracy; the former seems at least worth exploring.

13. Nussbaum MC. *Frontiers of justice: disability, nationality, species membership*, p. 213.

14. Nussbaum MC. *Frontiers of justice: disability, nationality, species membership*, pp. 180–95. As evidence of the dangers of the slippery slope, Nussbaum notes that persons with mental disabilities "are persistently treated as if they have no right to occupy public space" (199), and notes an instance in

which children with Down syndrome were denied admission to a zoo, for fear of upsetting the chimpanzees (199–200).

15. Nussbaum MC. *Frontiers of justice: disability, nationality, species membership*, pp. 190–3.

16. A white paper on bioethics and disabilities, circulated in advance of a conference on that subject held at Yeshiva University in January, 2007, listed ten areas of intersection between bioethics and disabilities studies. I am grateful to the authors, Adrienne Asch, Jeffrey Blustein, and David Wasserman, for that document, which at this writing is not available for public distribution.

17. Asch A. Recognizing death while affirming life: can end of life reform uphold a disabled person's interest in continued life? *Hastings Cent Rep* 35(6):S31–S36, 2005. Asch, for example, refuses to join the more extreme disabilities advocates who argued that the discontinuation of Terri Schiavo's feeding tube amounted to unjust discrimination against a person with a disability, and accepts that the diagnosis of persistent vegetative state in the Schiavo case was sufficiently proven.

18. Miller BL. Autonomy and the refusal of lifesaving treatment. *Hastings Cent Rep* 11(4):22–8, 1981.

19. Bouvia, a woman in her twenties with cerebral palsy and painful arthritis, checked herself into the hospital in Riverside, California in 1983. She requested that she be allowed to die by refusing any artificial feeding, and that the hospital administer appropriate pain management to keep her comfortable during the dying process. The eventual court ruling on her petition was that she had no right to force the hospital staff to assist in her suicide, and that the staff could legally insert a nasogastric tube and feed her against her wishes. Bioethicists generally objected to the court ruling that Bouvia could be force-fed contrary to her (apparently competently) expressed wishes; see, for example, Annas GJ. When suicide prevention becomes brutality: the case of Elizabeth Bouvia. *Hastings Cent Rep* 14(2):202–1, 1984; Kane FI. Keeping Elizabeth Bouvia alive for the public good. *Hastings Cent Rep* 15(6): 5–8, 1985. The life of Elizabeth Bouvia subsequently became very convoluted, and involved at least one more set of court rulings and medical attention at several different facilities. It seems reasonable, however, in hindsight to attribute her suicidal ideas in 1983 to a combination of a recent failed relationship, untreated depression, and inadequately treated pain. Later events suggested that Bouvia's expressed desire to die waned when those problems were adequately addressed.

20. During the 1980s, colleagues and I were called "Nazis" by local disabilities advocates, merely (as far as we could tell) for organizing conferences on the topic of rationing health care, and for suggesting that health-care resources were finite.

21. Daniels relies heavily on Rawls's theory of justice, and ties a right to health care to Rawls's principle of justice calling for equal opportunities. Daniels thinks this is plausible because in his lexical ordering of the principles of justice, Rawls places equal opportunity below the most basic

political rights, but above the principle that governs the distribution of economic goods. See, generally, Daniels N. *Just health care*. New York: Cambridge University Press, 1985. By Daniels's schema, if health care cannot restore an individual to something like "normal" functioning for the species, it cannot serve the goal of equal opportunity, and so justice cannot require that the care be provided.

22. One *foreseen* contingency is that with the development of new technologies, the cost of "adequate" assistance would inevitably increase in the future, analogous to increases in health-care costs due to the development of new technologies. I relegate this problem to the long list of practical issues that would have to be addressed if we were talking about actually implementing an entitlement program, as opposed to doing a conceptual analysis for ethical purposes.

23. In the next chapter, I will argue, in relation to questions of international justice, that there are times when a too-facile agreement with the general concept that "resources are finite" might serve to cloak unjust social arrangements. Specifically, I will question the requirement that programs to assist the health problems of developing countries must be "sustainable." At one level, "sustainable" may simply be a recognition of realistic resource limits; on another level. "sustainable" may be a disguised way of saying that resources are limited today because of social structures that favor a particular group in power, and we do not wish to threaten that group's privileged position. To me, however, it seems a far cry from concluding that *sometimes* invoking the finite-resources claim too quickly may perpetuate injustice, to concluding that *therefore* we should start with the assumption that *no* limits ought to be placed on available resources, for purposes of ethical argument.

# 10 ⁚⁚

# Environmental and Global Issues

At first sight, the two general topic areas combined in this chapter, environmental issues and globalization and international justice, might seem an illogical alliance. The latter might be linked conceptually to the general model that I derived from feminist ethics and described in Chapter 6. We can imagine the population of the developed world, and that of the developing world, standing next to each other in the one-up/one-down power relationship and therefore seeing a number of ethical issues quite differently. Listening to the voices of the one-down group might prove ethically insightful for the rest of us. By contrast, it is not clear how that model could apply to environmental issues.

Seen another way, the two matters may be more closely affiliated than first appearances suggest. If we return to the so-called "African way" of ethics as described by Godfrey Tangwa that we encountered in Chapter 7, we can see that that approach to ethics might cover both issues comfortably.[1] Speaking very generally, we are being called upon to expand the network of affiliations and the network of well-being that is necessary for optimal human flourishing. First, we learn that the individual human being cannot be in a good state of affairs if the family or clan is suffering. Ultimately we are challenged to see the "family" in this case as all of humankind. Next, we are confronted with the reality that our well-being is intimately connected with that of our environment. If the environment is degraded, our lives, our futures, and our children's existence are all threatened. This chapter will ask, very briefly, how bioethics might be different if it took these matters to be central to its task—starting with the environment.

## ⠭ The Potter Tradition in Bioethics

Two people more or less simultaneously coined the term "bioethics" in 1970–1971. A struggle for primacy ensued—whose version of bio-ethics would become the dominant definition of this new field? One group—not surprisingly, the better funded—won. Today, a small group of critics of mainstream bioethics contend that the only sound way for us to embrace our future is to rediscover and deepen the "losing" version.

In Madison, Wisconsin, Van Rensselaer Potter, a cancer biochemist, was pondering the deep philosophical questions at the intersections among human values, science and technology, and ecological threats to human survival. Searching for a term to describe his enterprise, he eventually hit on "bioethics," which became the title of the 1971 book that laid out his project.[2]

Meanwhile, in Washington, D.C., Andre Hellegers, an obstetrician-gynecologist with an interest in ethical issues, was meeting with Sargent and Eunice Kennedy Shriver about the new institute that they proposed to create at Georgetown University. The Shrivers, out of their concerns for those with mental disabilities, had become generally interested in medical ethics, with a special focus on reproductive ethics. From these discussions the term "bioethics" emerged as a possible name for what the new institute would address.

By "bioethics," Potter meant the questions about humankind's relationship with its environment, and the survival of the human species in the face of environmental threats such as pollution, overpopulation, and nuclear war. By "bioethics," Hellegers and his colleagues at Georgetown's new Kennedy Institute of Ethics meant something much narrower—the ethical questions that arose out of the practice of medicine, and out of research in the biological sciences.

One of the major projects undertaken by the Kennedy Institute in its first decade was the preparation of a four-volume *Encyclopedia of Bioethics*.[3] The triumph of the Hellegers-Kennedy sense of "bioethics" over the Potter sense was demonstrated by the absence of any entry by Potter, or about Potter's work, in the *Encyclopedia*. The injustice of this exclusion was later acknowledged and remedied; but allowing Potter a page or two in the *Encyclopedia* could not reverse the fact that the vast majority of those then working in bioethics adopted the Hellegers-Kennedy view of what they were about.[4]

In hindsight, Potter was destined to lose this battle, funding matters aside. Potter had no formal training in philosophical or theological ethics, and the main philosophical inspiration for his work was the renegade Jesuit writer Pierre Teilhard de Chardin, a figure whom most mainstream American intellectuals regarded with suspicion. Potter's writing was not in the language of ethics, as mainstream philosophical or theological ethicists would recognize it. It was easy to assume that Potter was a scientist who had wandered into an area where he was simply out of his depth. His call for a scientific ethic seemed to most analytic philosophers a simple violation of the fact–value distinction, and not worth their time or attention.[5]

This dismissal of Potter split bioethics off from an important tradition Potter represented. Potter was also influenced heavily by Aldo Leopold, one of the major figures in the early ecology movement in the United States. Potter later modified his preferred term to "global bioethics," by which he meant, briefly, the ethics of the biosphere, and explicitly linked that idea to the "Leopold legacy."[6] Peter J. Whitehouse argues that if today, bioethics were to rediscover the Potter-Leopold line of thought, we would be led to pay considerably more attention to:

- the future of environmental ethics
- the social aspects of environment
- nature-based spirituality and "deep ecology"
- the healing power of nature; and
- the ethics of public health.[7]

*An ecological bioethics?* Following Hurricane Katrina and the destruction of much of the city of New Orleans, including its health-care infrastructure, Jonathan Moreno sketched a possible bioethical approach to examining this catastrophe. For Moreno, the only possible way for us to do justice to the event is explicitly to dedicate ourselves to reviving the Potter school of global bioethics.[8]

For Moreno, what happened in Katrina is very clear. Three catastrophes occurred—the hurricane itself; the breaching of the levees after the hurricane had passed; and the failure of government institutions at all levels to provide effective security and aid in the aftermath. The roots of these catastrophes stretched well into the past. The infrastructure that would have made the institutions capable of responding well had been chronically neglected and underfunded, in part due to the general failure of the U.S. health-care system to take public health seriously. The geology of New Orleans and the ecology of the Gulf of Mexico had been gradually altered, removing all of the buffers that would, in years past, have helped to shelter the city from the hurricane and the storm surge. These alterations of the environment occurred because self-interest and economic development were given priority over the public interest and environmental protection—Moreno specifically blames the energy, gambling, and real-estate interests for their role.

The response to Katrina divided neatly along lines of social class and privilege. Those with automobiles and with means received timely warning and were able to flee. Those without such means were left behind and forced to endure the squalor of the inadequate shelters and the fear of a lawless city. Later, those who had been dependent on public housing found their neighborhoods the last to be reopened to habitation or to undergo repair, leading some to conclude that the black underclass was being treated as unwanted and expendable. Moreno contemplates all this and wonders about the role of bioethics. Since Katrina represents a generalized failure of our institutions, the institution of bioethics is also implicated. Moreno wonders if bioethics added to the failure in part because it had become a tool of privilege. The cutting-edge technological issues that bioethicists love to debate, such as embryonic stem cells and genetic engineering, belong to the wealthy. These issues are irrelevant to those around the globe who lack basic health care and public health. American institutions treated Katrina survivors in New Orleans and many surrounding areas about as we would have expected survivors to be treated in poor developing countries, so the notion of solidarity between the residents of those countries and the Katrina survivors (and their neglect by bioethics) seems apt.

Bioethics is supposed to be an intellectual discipline, so Moreno wonders why there has been so little exchange and cross-fertilization between bioethics and environmental ethics. He suggests that such cross-fertilization, besides invigorating both fields, might also help to mend fences in bioethics' political divisions post-Schiavo:

> While conservative and liberal thinkers might continue to disagree about familiar ethical issues like suitable limits on enhancement technologies, they should find common cause in the need to care for a fragile and increasingly ailing planet. In some ways, such a discourse would return us to the insight that gave rise to both fields [bioethics and ecology]—namely,

that human happiness and well-being is dependent upon a complex ecological system in which we are all inextricably linked, a system in which we are all actors and patients, doers and sufferers. We ignore these brute facts at our peril.[9]

One may certainly quibble with some of the specifics in Moreno's list of sins. He states, for example, that bioethics has done precious little to promote the cause of universal access to health care since the President's Commission report in the early 1980s. I believe that enough bioethicists have written enough books and articles about access to health care— including an active role in the ill-fated Clinton health-care reform effort of 1993–4—to rebut that accusation. But on the main point, the general failure to consider the bioethical implications of our relationship with the environment, I believe that Moreno is correct.

*An activist agenda for ecological bioethics?* We could imagine a number of levels at which bioethics might move toward a greater engagement with environmental issues. One relatively minimal connection would be to consider the human health consequences of ecological change. To return to the Katrina example, the residents of New Orleans spent several days wading through waist-deep water, that was full of petro-chemicals, raw sewage, and numerous pollutants. It is astounding that a more serious epidemic did not befall them, in addition to the sporadic cases of infections that were reported.

Another relatively minimal approach would be to explore the environmental record of health-related facilities. Are hospitals and clinics built and run in an environmentally friendly way? What would be the impact on the surrounding community if the local health-care institutions took the lead in setting the eco-friendly example?

A more expansive eco-agenda would emerge from fully grasping the Moreno's basic point, that human beings will not remain ideally healthy and flourishing in a degraded environment. Environmentalism is therefore an extension of health care and a serious concern for bioethics. What practical steps should take priority?[10]

American bioethicists might first note the role that their country plays in the global environmental situation. The United States may not be the world's worst polluter, but for a nation of its size and influence it is setting one of the worst examples. The United Nations has been one of the most effective institutions in negotiating international agreements on environmental progress. The U.S. role of refusing to sign international treaties, refusing to recognize international criminal courts, and refusing to live up to its own obligations to the U.N. very likely will have to change before real progress can occur.[11]

Another matter worthy of attention is the relatively low price tag associated with some important environmental advances. James Speth, for instance, calculates what it would cost to secure and manage approximately 15 percent of the world's total land area as a set of nature preserves, protecting regional biodiversity. The additional cost, he concludes, would be approximately $25 billion, which happens to be about what the wealthy countries of the world spend annually for pet food.[12]

Speth argues further that we will, in the end, not see much improvement in the global ecosystem until we make a concerted effort to end global poverty. Affluent nations usually have a choice about degrading the environment and destroying non-renewable resources; poor nations usually have no such choice. The need to attack global poverty as a tool for preserving the environment takes us directly to questions of globalization and international justice.

## ❡ Bioethics, Globalization, and Economic Development

Bioethics has run up against globalization and issues around economic development in poor nations in several contexts, apart from the environmental issues we have just been discussing.[13] Some of these, such as problems concerning cross-cultural ethical relativity and the controversy around female genital mutilation, we have already addressed in Chapter 7. Matters that we still need to address include questions about the costs of doing research trials in developing countries, and what obligations to improve the health of the local population conducting such trials places on investigators from the developed nations. As bioethics has turned to emerging infectious diseases and public health, we have also had to face questions about the prevention of diseases like SARS and avian influenza in the developing world, both for the benefit of the local communities and also for prevention of worldwide pandemics.

Are issues such as these best addressed one at a time? Or is there an overarching concept of globalization, economic development, and international justice that ought to guide us in this area generally? I will here defend the theory of justice that we encountered in the chapter on disabilities, the capabilities approach, and related theories of international obligations, drawing on the work of Amartya Sen and Martha Nussbaum.

Nussbaum, as we have seen, argues that of the various theories of social justice growing out of the social contract tradition, the deepest and overall most satisfactory is John Rawls's theory of "justice as fairness."[14] Rawls derived his theory both from social-contract theory and from Kantian ethics.[15] For our present purposes, the most important social-contract lesson from Rawls is the idea that the basic structure of and rules for society ought to be those that the parties most involved, with the proper information and in the appropriate circumstances, would freely assent to. The major Kantian element is the basic worth and dignity of the individual, ruling out crude utilitarian proposals by which the rights of the few are sacrificed for the general well-being of the many.

Rawls, however, made it very clear initially that he intended justice-as-fairness to remain within national boundaries, and specifically to apply to a nation with a well-established liberal tradition and with reasonable material affluence, such as the United States.[16] Sen and Nussbaum, in developing their own theories of international justice, see themselves as extending and refining, rather than rejecting, Rawls's most basic and important ideas.[17]

Let us start with something we have already reviewed, Nussbaum's list of ten capabilities that are central to human dignity.[18]

- A reasonable life span
- Bodily health
- Bodily integrity and safety
- Being able to use one's senses, to imagine, think, and reason
- Being able to experience the range of human emotions
- Practical reasoning, the ability to plan one's life
- Engaging in social affiliations and interactions
- Living in the world of nature in fellowship with other plant and animal species
- Opportunities to play and to enjoy leisure
- Reasonable control over one's political and material environment, including rights to political participation

Previously, we used this list to address the duties that our society owed to persons with disabilities. Nussbaum proposes that we use the same list to determine what basic capabilities ought to be protected and supported by all nations for their peoples. Where nations lack the economic resources to provide threshold amounts of these basic capabilities to their population, we must then ask whether justice requires that wealthier nations step in to contribute those resources.[19]

One immediate objection to any redistributive argument from justice is that it is not the fault of the wealthy nations that the developing countries lack resources, so the wealthy should have no obligation to donate resources. This is perhaps analogous to an argument regarding persons with disabilities, that the able-bodied did not cause their impairments, so that it would be unjust to tax the able-bodied to provide more assistive services. To meet that objection it was necessary to introduce the social-construction model of disability, showing that disability, properly understood, is caused by certain social arrangements and decisions, rather than solely by physical impairments. The able-bodied participate in making those decisions and benefit from those social arrangements. They therefore cannot evade moral responsibility.

With regard to the plight of the developing nations, it is relatively easier to connect the dots and to see that the wealthy nations are not blameless with regard to the former's lack of resources. We can see (though I will not devote the space here to documenting the case) how historical colonial patterns of exploitation robbed those countries of resources to benefit the wealthy nations, and how many international trade and business arrangements today perpetuate that pattern of exploitation. In any event, I will assume for purposes of argument that there is some level of responsibility among the nations of the developed world for the current status of the developing world.

The next objection one might encounter is that any redistributive proposal based on the capabilities list amounts to cultural imperialism or neocolonialism, an attempt to force a Western world-view on all people and cultures. Nussbaum replies that her list of ten capabilities is quite reasonably seen as universally acceptable because it is open-ended in the correct way. Different cultures will disagree strenuously about how to define or characterize each of the ten capabilities—what, for example, counts as adequate housing, or what the content of education ought to be. But Nussbaum doubts that we will encounter many cultures that would simply reject out of hand even a few out of the list of ten.[20] Sen adds, "The culturally fearful often take a very fragile view of each culture and tend to underestimate our ability to learn from elsewhere without being overwhelmed by that experience."[21] Sen argues that when it comes to deciding whether to extend human capabilities and freedoms or to hold fast to traditional cultural mores, "different sections of the society (and not just the socially privileged) should be able to be active in the decisions regarding what to preserve and what to let go. There is no compulsion to preserve every departing lifestyle even at heavy cost, but there is a real need—for social justice—for people to be able to take part in these social decisions, if they so choose."[22] If the people affected by such decisions ought to be able to choose their own fate, that drives home the importance of the capabilities of basic literacy, freedom of information, and rights of democratic participation. Sen and Nussbaum require that such capabilities be viewed as universal human rights, and Nussbaum explicitly links her own version of the capabilities approach to a human rights philosophy.[23]

Sen aims his arguments particularly at those who argue that, for developing nations, economic development must precede any concern about wider human rights or capabilities—"that focusing on democracy and political liberty is a luxury that a poor country 'cannot afford.'"[24] He defends the position that:

> [E]xpansion of freedom is viewed as both (1) the *primary end* and (2) the *principal means* of development. They can be called respectively the "constitutive role" and the "instrumental role" of freedom in development. The constitutive role of freedom relates to the importance of substantive freedom in enriching human life. The substantive freedoms include elementary capabilities like being able to avoid such deprivations as starvation, undernourishment, escapable morbidity and premature mortality, as well as the freedoms that are associated with being literate and numerate, enjoying political participation and uncensored speech and so on....Development, in this view, is the process of expanding human freedoms....[25]

Sen gives a number of examples from the history of Asia during the twentieth century. He argues that, in general, when a poor country has public policies that favor basic education and health care, and then undergoes economic growth, one quickly sees expansion of social opportunities, reduction in mortality rates, and increased life expectancy, among other general social benefits. By contrast, when countries without a basic social commitment to rights and capabilities undergo economic growth, such benefits are seen much more slowly, if at all, even though gross domestic product per capita rises.[26] In these latter countries, wealth may flow to the hands of a privileged class, but the vast majority of the population remains uneducated, unhealthy, and vulnerable to a range of woes and miseries. In short, the engine for further economic development is not constructed. In contrast, in the former countries that took care from the beginning to secure the benefits of an educated and healthy population, economic growth builds upon itself much faster and spreads much more widely through the country due to those favorable conditions.

Suppose that the leaders of a wealthy nation are reading over our shoulders, and decide that, as a matter of justice, they should provide increased aid to poorer nations. What form should that aid take? Sen argues, in keeping with his historical analysis, that the wealthy nation would be best advised to invest in the education and health infrastructures. There are two reasons for this. The first, already noted, is that the basic capabilities and freedoms, including education and health, are important drivers of, or play an instrumental role, in economic development. The second is a matter of efficiency. Education and health care are personnel-heavy sectors of the economy. Most of the money invested there goes to the costs of labor. In a low-wage economy typical for a developing nation, a relatively small investment from a wealthy nation buys a lot of education or health care.[27]

Why is any of this a concern for bioethics? Nussbaum sketches a picture that draws on philosophical traditions going back to the ancient Stoics, Aristotle, Cicero, and the natural law theories of Hugo Grotius— that we are by our nature beings that seek a common good and wish to live a life of sociability, in keeping with our native intelligence:

> This intelligence is a moral intelligence. The three central facts about human beings that this moral intelligence apprehends are the dignity of the human being as an ethical being, a dignity that is fully equal no matter where humans are placed; human sociability, which means that part of a life with human dignity is a common life with others organized so as to respect that equal dignity; and the multiple facts of human need, which suggest that this common life must do something for us all, fulfilling needs up to a point at which human dignity is not undermined by hunger, or violent assault, or unequal treatment in the political realm. Combining the fact of sociability with the other two facts, we arrive at the idea that a central part of our own good…is to produce, and live in, a world that is morally decent, a world in which all human beings have what they need to live a life worthy of human dignity.[28]

"The capabilities approach," Nussbaum continues, "is an oriented approach that supplies a partial account of basi In other words, it says that a world in which people ities on the list is a minimally just and decent w

This core philosophical conception leads to a set of practical principles for global structures and relationships:

1. The presence of an international responsibility to secure basic capabilities does not relieve the responsibility of domestic institutions. Developing world nations cannot persist in their own exploitations of their own population, through government corruption, for example, based on the argument that their problems are all the fault of the wealthy nations and they should fix them.
2. We should respect national sovereignty within the constraints of the basic capabilities and human rights.
3. Prosperous nations have responsibility to transfer substantial amounts of wealth to poorer nations.
4. Multinational corporations have analogous responsibilities for regions where they operate.
5. International institutions such as the International Monetary Fund must be designed to be fair to poor and developing countries.
6. We need a thin, decentralized, but still forceful global apparatus, such as a reformed and invigorated United Nations. (The dangers of global tyranny argue against excessive centralization of power.)
7. All institutions and most individuals should focus on the problems of the disadvantaged in each region.
8. Prominent duties include care for the ill, elderly, children, and disabled.
9. The family should be treated as precious but not private. Abuse of women, for example, should not be allowed simply because it occurs within the "privacy" of the home.
10. We have a special obligation to support education as a key to the empowerment of those now disadvantaged.[30]

Will a conception of international justice in keeping with such a list of practical principles lead to a wave of strife, and neocolonial intrusions of the Western nations into the affairs of other countries? We need to return here to a point we addressed in discussing multicultural issues. The fact that the current practices of a certain nation fall short of our concept of international justice does not give us a moral warrant to intervene in the affairs of that nation. In extreme cases, gross violation of basic human rights on a widespread scale demand international intervention, as was the case in Rwanda and Bosnia, and is the case as of this writing in Sudan. In the vast majority of disputes over international justice, Principle #2, calling for respect for national sovereignty, holds priority. Nussbaum argues, following Grotius, that one of the basic goods of human sociality is our ability to join with others to give laws to the collective in which all of us live. In most circumstances, the nation-state is the only structural way to accomplish this good. It is therefore a basic good to human beings that we are able to live within sovereign nations, however imperfect (up to a point) other nations may think those to be. Respect for human dignity requires at least some degree of respect for national sovereignty. In sum, we should rely not on military intervention to enforce international justice in most cases, but rather on the carrot of economic aid combined with the stick of aggressive diplomacy.[31]

Physician-anthropologist Paul Farmer works to provide health care in rural Haiti to communities that have been seriously disadvantaged by what he terms the "structural violence" of a new hydroelectric dam. The dam destroyed the lands the people used to farm, giving them back in return neither water nor electricity, while the Haitian urban elite and foreign investors grow rich off the proceeds. From Farmer's vantage point, today's bioethics is a part of the problem—either we bioethicists ignore the issues in Haiti completely, or we give aid and comfort to the wealthy and powerful by defending such vague principles as "sustainability" and "cost-effectiveness." Farmer finds much more ethical wisdom in liberation theology, in defense of his work, than he does in contemporary bioethics.[32] While one could quibble at the margins about Farmer's anti-bioethics diatribe (and Farmer himself admits that he finds some promising developments within bioethics), I basically am in sympathy with his larger agenda. I believe that if bioethics gave central attention to a capabilities approach to international justice along the lines recommended by Sen and Nussbaum, then Farmer would no longer find very much to criticize.

## ⠴ Conclusions: An Internationally Just Bioethics

A bioethics enterprise that was fully informed by these concerns for global justice would resonate with several themes that have surfaced previously in our survey. We saw in Chapter 1 and elsewhere that several authors had accused bioethics of being insufficiently attentive to public health, population health, international health, and (as symptomatic of the above) infectious disease. All these issues would be on the front burner if bioethics took more seriously the health needs of the entire global community.

Another dimension of bioethics' purported neglect of global matters can best be addressed by looking at how we approach new technologies, the subject of the next chapter. Can the charge be sustained that, in large part because of our fascination with fancy, expensive new technologies, bioethics in the United States has "practiced 'rich man's ethics' "?[33] A discussion of how bioethics might most productively approach new technologies will provide additional opportunities to see how bioethics could better address issues of global justice.

NOTES TO CHAPTER 10

1. Tangwa GB. The traditional African perception of a person. Some implications for bioethics. *Hastings Cent Rep* 30(5):39–43, 2000.
2. Potter VR. *Bioethics: bridge to the future*. Englewood Cliffs, NJ: Prentice-Hall, 1971. Potter had used the term the previous year in a journal publication: Potter VR. Bioethics: the science of survival. *Perspect Biol Med* 14:127–53, 1970. A handy recent summary of Potter's work and influence is Whitehouse PJ. The rebirth of bioethics: extending the original formulations of Van Rensselaer Potter. *Am J Bioethics* 3(4):W26–W31, 2003.

    As I was completing work on this book, I learned of the writings of a German Protestant pastor, Fritz Jahr, who proposed the concept of "Bio-Ethik" in 1927 and in a subsequent series of publications. According to Sass, Jahr proposed extending Kant's categorical imperative to the animal and plant worlds, so that all living things ought to be treated as ends-in-themselves and never as means only, insofar as possible: Sass HM. Fritz Jahr's 1927 concept of bioethics. *Kennedy Inst Ethics J* 17:279–95, 2007. Jahr thus to some extent anticipated the Potter tradition in bioethics, but I see no evidence that Potter was aware of Jahr's work.
3. Reich WT (ed.) *Encyclopedia of bioethics* (4 vol.). New York: Free Press, 1978.
4. A later historical account of Potter's role, and his probable priority in coining the term "bioethics," from the editor of the first and second editions of the *Encyclopedia of Bioethics*, is Reich WT. The word "bioethics": its birth and the legacies of those who shaped it. *Kennedy Inst Ethics J* 4:319–35, 1994; Reich WT. The word "bioethics": the struggle over its earliest meanings. *Kennedy Inst Ethics J* 5:19–34, 1995.
5. My own career in bioethics somewhat illustrates Potter's fate. Potter's 1971 volume, *Bioethics*, was actually one of the first books on the subject that I read, since my undergraduate mentor at Michigan State University, James E. Trosko, a molecular biologist, had been a student of Potter's and arranged several times for Potter to speak at Michigan State (and for a later volume of Potter's on bioethics to be published by Michigan State University Press). When I wrote my first book on bioethics, *Ethical Decisions in Medicine* (Boston: Little, Brown, 1976) I included a sympathetic

mention of Potter's views. When I began formal graduate study of philosophy in 1973, I came to embrace the analytic school then dominant in Anglo-American philosophy, and found it harder and harder to translate any of Potter's views into the language of ethics that I was then learning. Eventually references to Potter dropped out of my own work, although I continued to admire him as a person. Whitehouse similarly extols Potter for his personal virtue and authenticity; Whitehouse PJ. The rebirth of bioethics: extending the original formulations of Van Rensselaer Potter. *Am J Bioethics* 3(4):W26–W31, 2003.

6. Potter VR. *Global bioethics: building on the Leopold legacy.* East Lansing, MI: Michigan State University Press, 1988.

7. Whitehouse PJ. The rebirth of bioethics: extending the original formulations of Van Rensselaer Potter. *Am J Bioethics* 3(4):W26–W31, 2003.

8. Moreno JD. In the wake of Katrina: has "bioethics" failed? *Am J Bioethics* 5(5):W18–W19, 2005. Moreno even goes as far as to note that the dykes in The Netherlands are designed to withstand much worse stress than were the New Orleans levees, adding, "who better to appreciate the delicate balance of nature, exemplified by land reclaimed from the sea, than a Dutchman?" (referring to Potter's Dutch ancestry).

9. Moreno JD. In the wake of Katrina: has "bioethics" failed?

10. In a book such as this I am not able to survey all the current literature on the environment. I have chosen to use one source; Speth JG. *Red sky at morning: America and the crisis of the global environment.* New Haven, CT: Yale University Press, 2005. I am grateful to Karin Ewer for research assistance.

11. Speth JG. *Red sky at morning: America and the crisis of the global environment,* p. 111.

12. Speth JG. *Red sky at morning: America and the crisis of the global environment,* p. 42.

13. Nancy Kass offers a history of bioethics' gradual incorporation of issues of global justice, situated within that part of bioethics that addresses ethical issues in public health. She argues that public health bioethics entered a new era around the beginning of the twenty-first century, and situates global justice issues as a part of that unfolding development; Kass NE. Public health ethics: from foundations and frameworks to justice and global public health. *J Law Med Ethics* 32:232–42, 2004.

14. Rawls J. *A theory of justice.* Cambridge, MA: Belknap Press of Harvard University Press, 1971; Rawls J. *Political liberalism.* New York: Columbia University Press, 1993; Rawls J. *Justice as fairness: a restatement.* Cambridge, MA: Belknap Press of Harvard University Press, 2001.

15. Some of us who are not Kantian scholars may have forgotten that Kant, in matters of social and international justice, also situated himself within the social contract tradition; Nussbaum M. *Frontiers of justice: disability, nationality, species membership.* Cambridge, MA: Belknap Press of Harvard University Press, 2006, pp. 50–2.

16. In his late writings, Rawls made some attempt to extend his theory of justice internationally, most prominently in Rawls J. *The law of peoples:*

*with the idea of public reason revisited.* Cambridge, MA: Harvard University Press, 1999. Nussbaum argues that these attempts are ultimately limited and unsatisfactory: Nussbaum M. *Frontiers of justice: disability, nationality, species membership*, pp. 238–70.

17. Sen A. *Development as freedom.* New York, Anchor Books, 2000, p. 74; Nussbaum M. *Frontiers of justice: disability, nationality, species membership*, pp. 22–25. I regard one of Rawls's most important contributions to theories of justice his "Difference Principle," regarding distributive justice in income and wealth. I therefore find it a matter of concern that Nussbaum's capabilities approach requires that we bracket the Difference Principle to one side, if not that we reject it entirely: Nussbaum M. *Frontiers of justice: disability, nationality, species membership*, pp. 56–67. My concerns about these implications take us well beyond the scope of this book, however, as they apply more to justice within rather than between nations.

18. Nussbaum MC. *Frontiers of justice: disability, nationality, species membership*, pp. 76–78. Nussbaum draws her approach to capabilities largely from the work of Amartya Sen.

19. Nussbaum M. *Frontiers of justice: disability, nationality, species membership*, pp. 273–324.

20. Nussbaum M. *Frontiers of justice: disability, nationality, species membership*, pp. 295–8.

21. Sen A. *Development as freedom*, p. 243.

22. Sen A. *Development as freedom*, p. 242. Sen notes further that when we in the West talk about preserving the cultures of non-Western countries, we are often unduly deferential to those in power in those nations, as it is those in power who tend to be present in the international venues where such matters are discussed (247).

23. Nussbaum M. *Frontiers of justice: disability, nationality, species membership*, pp. 284–91. Paul Farmer and Nicole Gastineau Campos, criticizing today's bioethics for ignoring the problems of the sick poor in developing countries, call for bioethics to adopt a human rights perspective as an antidote: Farmer P, Campos NG. New malaise: bioethics and human rights in the global era. *J Law Med Ethics* 32:243–51, 2004.

    Griffin Trotter (in accusing bioethics of deeply-rooted leftist biases) and Tristram Engelhardt (in accusing bioethics of ignoring the robust moral pluralism of the world) would presumably both object to any reliance by bioethics on such supposed lists of universal human rights. I take it that the main objection is to a shell game where we imagine that we have "discovered" these universal human rights in the same way that a botanist discovers a new species of plant; and that bioethicists' consensus about these human rights is sufficient to establish their moral weight and heft. I see no problem with admitting, first, that any list of supposedly universal human rights will betray all sorts of political biases; and second, that doing anything useful with such a list of rights is a matter for protracted negotiation, not for a quick-and-dirty consensus among a group of academics. I fail to see how either admission weakens the case for a conception of justice such as Nussbaum and

Sen are making. On these debates, see Trotter G. Left bias in academic bioethics: three dogmas. In: Eckenwiler LA, Cohn FG, eds. *The ethics of bioethics: mapping the moral landscape.* Baltimore: Johns Hopkins University Press, 2007: 108–17; and Engelhardt HT. Bioethics as politics: a critical reassessment. In: Eckenwiler LA, Cohn FG, eds. *The ethics of bioethics: mapping the moral landscape.* Baltimore: Johns Hopkins University Press, 2007: 118–33.

24. Sen A. *Development as freedom*, p. 147.
25. Sen A. *Development as freedom*, p. 36.
26. Sen A. *Development as freedom*, p. 45.
27. Sen A. *Development as freedom*, pp. 47–8. Sen did not add here, but could have, that the diseases prevalent in the developing world are relatively cheap to prevent or treat compared to the "diseases of affluence" and chronic illnesses prevalent in the West. What is most needed is often public health and basic primary care at the nurse-practitioner level, as opposed to hospitals and specialists.
28. Nussbaum M. *Frontiers of justice: disability, nationality, species membership,* p. 274.
29. Nussbaum M. *Frontiers of justice: disability, nationality, species membership,* p. 274.
30. Nussbaum M. *Frontiers of justice: disability, nationality, species membership,* pp. 315–24.
31. Nussbaum M. *Frontiers of justice: disability, nationality, species membership,* pp. 255–62. Nussbaum takes issue with Rawls's "The Law of Peoples" because Rawls fails to explain just why nations have moral importance: Rawls J. *The law of peoples; with the idea of public reason revisited.* Cambridge, MA: Harvard University Press, 1999.
32. Farmer P. *Pathologies of power: health, human rights, and the new war on the poor.* Berkeley, CA: University of California Press, 2003.
33. "Here in the United States, our main bioethics societies, and bioethicists as individuals, have tended to concentrate on individualistic ethics and its problems (euthanasia, abortion, termination of care, IVF, etc.) and have, to a large measure, practiced 'rich man's ethics' "; Loewy EH. Bioethics: past, present, and an open future. *Camb Q Healthc Ethics* 11:388–97, 2002.

# 11 ::

# New Technologies

:: The "Hastings Mantra"

Those of us who became involved in bioethics in the 1970s heard a certain message repeated *ad nauseam.* It seemed to assume qualities of a ritualistically invoked mantra. As one of the two major bioethics think tanks dating from those days already has a mantra named after it, I will call this mantra the "Hastings mantra."[1]

The Hastings mantra has two parts:

- The development of novel medical technologies confronts us with ethical challenges of a sort never before encountered.
- It is vitally important that we address those emerging ethical challenges pro-actively, before the technology has come into widespread use. (The mantra seldom proceeds to answer the logical follow-up question, "Or else what?" since one cannot provide any very long list of technologies that were *not* put into use merely because pro-active bioethical analysis objected.)[2]

As often as the mantra has been mindlessly repeated, both clauses can be questioned. Paul Litton asks searching questions about the emergence of a new subfield, "nanoethics." He admits that new nanotechnologies are qualitatively different in some ways from other, older technologies. And he admits that they will pose important ethical questions, especially about safety and privacy. But he insists that with just a little thought, one can see important parallels between all of these ethical questions and the questions that have been raised in the past about other technologies. It is not at all clear that a new "nanoethics" must be constructed solely to address these ethical conundrums. Finally, Litton adds, there is no reason to imagine that pro-actively attacking the ethical problems will get us any farther than waiting on developments. Any pre-emptive ethics strikes will probably be based on incomplete facts about the technology and its likely uses. The likelihood of being flat-out wrong about some important fact probably outweighs any supposed advantages of getting one's ethical dibs in first.[3]

I will approach the relationship between bioethics and new technologies as an admitted skeptic, suggesting that what Litton says is true of nanotechnology, has in fact been true of many of the new technologies with which bioethics has had love affairs. New technologies do indeed raise important ethical issues, at least on occasion. But the path from the technology to ethical wisdom may have more twists and turns than is commonly appreciated.


## ⠴ Some Historical Case Studies

A few historical examples may help illustrate the various ways new technologies may have ethical implications, of perhaps unexpected sorts.

My first case study is taken from the treatment of cholera during the first epidemic of that disease (commonly termed "Asiatic cholera") in England in the early 1830s.[4] When cholera first appeared in Europe, some physicians judged it to be spread from person to person, but contagious theories soon gave way to the dominant miasmatic model then used to explain most febrile epidemic diseases. It was assumed that decaying organic matter in the environment gave rise to noxious gases, of unknown composition, which, in the right climatic conditions, could be spread through the atmosphere. Once breathed in, the miasma could cause disease. Which disease it caused (cholera, yellow fever, influenza, or malaria, for instance), as well as whether that individual got sick or remained healthy, was attributed to the person's constitutional predispositions as well as to the aforementioned climatic variables. It was assumed that the route of entry for these miasmata into the body was the respiratory tract; and to be spread to other parts of the body, the disease agent would necessarily traverse the bloodstream.

Most observers of the pathological changes caused by cholera agreed that as the disease progressed, the blood became progressively thicker, and that the watery components of the blood seemed to be lost. (Those who advocated bleeding as a treatment, in order to remove the noxious humors from the body, were often thwarted by the practical difficulty of getting the blood to flow.) The role that this change in the blood played in the overall disease process, and whether it provided any clues as to appropriate therapy, was nevertheless hotly disputed.

William Brooke O'Shaughnessy, who performed some pioneering chemical experiments on the blood of cholera victims and confirmed its state of dehydration, proposed in 1832 that injecting a saline solution into the veins ought to be an effective way of reversing the effects of the disease. Thomas Latta, a Scottish physician, took up O'Shaughnessy's proposal and put it to the practical test. He was able to treat a middle-aged woman, who initially had seemed nearly moribund, to a complete recovery using his injections. Other cases did not turn out so well, and Latta came under considerable criticism. George Johnson, writing in 1855, reviewed the case reports he could find of saline injections, concluding that of 156 cases, only 25 recovered. Johnson expressed the majority opinion when he concluded that the weight of the evidence was strongly against the use of injections.

It was not until the 1890s that interest in intravenous fluid therapy for cholera revived. Today, we believe that the dehydration, caused by the copious diarrhea produced by the cholera organism's effect on the lining of the intestine, is the major manifestation of the disease, and that the best possible therapy is prompt and massive rehydration—intravenously if necessary and if the proper equipment is available, or orally in other cases.

We can see in hindsight that, in one sense, O'Shaughnessy and Latta were completely correct in their proposed mode of treatment. In another sense it did not matter at all whether they were correct or not. It was all very well to propose, as a matter of theory, that restoring water to the blood would counteract the disease process. The technological tools of the day were almost wholly inadequate for the process of intravenous saline injection. No part of the typical intravenous apparatus of today—whether the container to hold the fluid, the connecting tubing, or the hollow needle suitable for intravenous insertion—was generally available or reliable in its function. In the absence of any modern knowledge of asepsis and infection, any widespread attempt at intravenous infusion would have caused great harm. (By contrast, oral rehydration therapy could well have succeeded in that environment, had anyone thought to employ it.)

The lesson I draw from this case study is the pedestrian one, that advances in medical theoretical understanding and advances in technology must proceed more or less hand in hand if the understanding is to have any effect on practical outcomes. Moreover (and perhaps less obvious), if one has the understanding but lacks the technology, it is not necessarily clear at the time what the problem is. I am not aware of any physician who wrote during the early cholera epidemics, "We have a great understanding of what we need to do to reverse the effects of cholera; the trouble is that we lack an effective technology to deliver the preferred treatment."[5] Sometimes technology feeds back into medical theory. It seems plausible to claim that today we think about the nature of cholera differently from our forebears of the nineteenth century, *in part because we know* that fluid-replacement technology can effectively reverse most of cholera's deleterious effects.

The next case study is the development of the clinical thermometer in the middle and later years of the nineteenth century.[6] To those of us who cut our bioethical teeth on respirators and artificial hearts, the thermometer may seem like small potatoes, but for its time it was a great technological breakthrough. Textbooks of medicine began to demonstrate their up-to-dateness by including fever charts. The patient's hospital record was no longer the completely narrative compendium it had been previously—perhaps the first in a long series of steps that transformed the hospital chart into primarily a repository of quantitative data.

For all its dramatic possibilities, the clinical thermometer ended up making modest differences in diagnostic accuracy and little difference in treatment. Its development occurred at about the same time as the major advances in bacteriology that soon overshadowed it. Being able to determine what microbe caused a particular disease led, in the long run, to more solid advances in diagnosis and treatment than did one's ability to construct an elegant, hour-by-hour fever curve.

The clinical thermometer had perhaps its greatest impact on the relations between the physician and nurse. According to the old medicine, a fever was a qualitative phenomenon that had to be described precisely by an expert. Only a properly trained physician could be trusted with the task of observing and reporting the nature of the fever, just as only the physician could sound the lungs with the stethoscope and report the findings.[7]

With the advent of the clinical thermometer, all of the complex description of the fever was suddenly reduced to two numbers—the degrees according to thermometer, and the time of day at which the measurement was taken.[8] It seemed obvious that one did not need a physician's training to read these two numbers and to write the results down. At first, jealous physicians set rules that forbade nurses to read the thermometer, but that obvious rear-guard action was soon abandoned. The result, viewed negatively, was one of the first chinks in the physician's authority over the sickroom; or viewed positively, one of the first steps toward the creation of a true team of professional caregivers.[9]

The lesson that I draw from the thermometer case study is that the most significant repercussions of a new technology might be its effect on social relationships and social networks. And this effect of a new technology might be especially difficult to predict.

The final case study is drawn from Joel Howell's study of technology in American hospitals between 1900 and 1920. Howell is interested in the rate of uptake of x-rays and of simple laboratory tests such as urinalysis and blood counts. He notes that if one reviews hospital charts from 1900, one sees very few such data recorded, even in patients where there is a clear medical indication. The story is quite different in 1920 when the vast majority of patients for whom these tests would be suitable have results recorded.[10]

Howell then tries to puzzle out what accounts for this change, and determines that it has virtually nothing to do with the actual x-ray or laboratory equipment. One cause is the way that work in the hospital was conceived of. A major revolution in hospital management occurred within that twenty-year period. "Efficiency experts" had turned to the well-run American factory as their model for all organizations, and hospital managers had eagerly bought into this industrial model of efficiency. As a consequence, important new machines showed up in hospitals between 1900 and 1910, but these were not medical machines per se, and they did not show up in the areas devoted to patient care. They were typewriters and adding machines. Along with the advent of these tools of industrial efficiency, and a cadre of managers who knew what to do with them and who depended on them, came the technological change that probably had the most to do with the rapid uptake of the "new technologies" of x-ray and clinical laboratory—the development and extensive use of preprinted forms for inserting the resulting data into the hospital chart.[11]

Howell's thoughtful analysis suggests several lessons. First, new technologies are not isolated creations; they nest within systems of thought and activity. One can completely misunderstand them by locating them within the wrong system. Earlier medical historians looking, for instance, at the history of radiology probably thought that what happened in the office of the hospital manager was totally irrelevant to the *clinical* use of the new x-ray machines, except perhaps for the basic decision of whether or not to buy the machine. Howell gained his insights by seeing that these machines were also located within the larger system of industrial efficiency and the revolution in hospital management. Second, one can easily look at the technology that matters less and ignore the technology that matters more. A preprinted piece of paper stuck in a hospital chart might not seem like a "new technology" at all. The typewriter (which the newly organized radiology department used to enter the data from its test on the pre-printed form, in the proper "modern" format) might not seem like a new *medical* technology. Yet both were ultimately more important in deciding what happened in the hospital and in the care of patients than the cathode ray tube itself, which stood in a corner gathering dust in 1905, but which was in constant use in 1920.

My main point in going over these historical case studies is to argue that when confronting a new medical technology with the goal of elucidating the bioethical issues, it is quite easy to ask a lot of misguided questions and to miss the questions that matter most. I do not want to insist that all attempts to front-load the ethical analysis will necessarily be futile, and that only historical hindsight will suffice to throw the issues into their proper perspective. I do suggest, however, that whenever we have come to ethical conclusions in advance of the application of a new technology, we will almost certainly need later to revisit and often revise those conclusions.


## ✷  A More Recent Case Study: IVF

There were no bioethicists about to analyze cholera treatment in 1832, or clinical thermometers in 1868, or x-ray machines in 1900. There were bioethicists around when in vitro fertilization (IVF) was undergoing its developmental stages in the 1970s. How did we do? We ended up looking silly—twice.

The first silliness occurred when a number of bioethics thinkers, mostly of what today would be called a conservative bent, issued dire warnings about the consequences of IVF. Clearly, if these thinkers had had the power to stop IVF in its tracks, they would have done so without hesitation. The notion of "test tube babies" suggested striking analogies with Aldous Huxley's dystopian novel *Brave New World*, and perhaps in hindsight that powerful literary imagery addled the bioethicists' brains. Grim forecasts appeared of the cultural Rubicon that was about to be crossed. We would go from having our children in the "natural" way to "manufacturing" our offspring. A loving, caring, and above all else *human* relationship would be replaced with a cold, artificial, mechanical relationship.[12] In the old mode of parenting, humans accepted their children as God's gifts, the imperfect along with the rest. (Apparently none of these bioethicists had ever attended a Little League game and watched the behavior of parents along the sidelines.) The bad new mode of parenting would generate a relentless demand that the products of manufacture must be perfect, so we would engineer the intelligence, physical appearance, and any other aspect of the child we could get our technological hands on.

In 1978, Louise Brown was born in England, the first child to result from IVF. Some commentators had *almost* gone as far as to wish that the first such infant would be born with two heads or with no arms, or in some other way be a monstrosity. They admitted that wishing such an outcome on an innocent child was hardly ethically sound. But they predicted (probably correctly) that if such were the outcome, the immediate public revulsion would probably quickly destroy any further support for IVF, no matter what its actual scientific potential.[13] To the disappointment of anyone who actually thought that way, Louise Brown was quite a normal and indeed unremarkable infant. Today she is a normal and quite unremarkable young woman, as the media rediscover when an anniversary rolls around and they are moved to look her up.

Today, IVF is almost completely a ho-hum technology. None of the dire predictions seems to have come true.[14] Our society may, morally, have gone straight to hell since 1978, but it seems quite implausible to single out IVF as the root cause of this collapse. In hindsight, the dire predictions mostly had to do with the relationships between parents and children. IVF allowed many people who could not otherwise have genetically related children to do so. Once those children were born, the parents related to them pretty much in the same way that all parents relate to their children. The IVF technology by itself seemed in hindsight to be powerless to foster all the changes that were predicted. The willingness of some bioethicists to go out on a limb and insist that the sky would fall if IVF were embraced counts as the first episode of silliness.

The second silliness occurred twenty years later when we came to debate human cloning. I wish immediately to go on record as being opposed to human reproductive cloning, and I believe that there are excellent reasons (unlike the IVF case) to prohibit it. The ethical concerns have to do primarily with the high mortality and morbidity rates attached to existing cloning technologies, coupled with the lack of any corresponding benefit from cloning used as a reproductive technology. (The benefits that have occasionally been claimed for cloning mostly indicate a misunderstanding of the true nature of cloning and the resulting individual human being, such as the idea that parents losing a child could somehow clone a "carbon copy" as a "replacement.")[15]

Arguing against human reproductive cloning on ethical grounds, therefore, is hardly silly. What is silly, however, is trotting out the *very same dire predictions that were raised in the IVF case, without any acknowledgment that when applied to that earlier technology, these predictions proved baseless.* At the very least, one should be called upon to explain why human cloning is quite different from IVF, such that we could be so wrong back then, but right today. Yet most of these bioethicists (despite in a few cases being the very same people) wrote about human cloning as if we had a collective amnesia for the voluminous literature on IVF.

These "manufactured baby" attacks on the ethics of cloning were not only silly, they were also mean. Passions back in the 1970s had led some bioethicists to go as far as *almost* to wish for the birth of deformed babies. Similarly inflamed passions during the cloning debate led bioethicists to level the charge of inhumanity, not at the cloning technology, but *at the infant* who would be born as the result of the cloning experiment. This infant, it would claimed, would be morally defective; unlike the rest of us in a very important way—and this charge was leveled against a baby whose only crime was to stand (through no act of its own) in the same genetic relationship to another human being as an identical twin. As James Rachels warned in another context, when bioethicists go into tsk-tsk, finger-wagging mode in response to whatever was the latest headline on the evening news, do not expect anything very wise or insightful to result.[16]

## ⠱ Bioethics and New Technologies: General Observations

Can anything usefully be said, in general, about the way bioethics ought to approach the issues raised by new technological developments?

Exactly what is the posture of bioethics toward new technologies? We have seen how Rachels scolded bioethicists for resorting to finger-wagging criticism as their default mode when faced with some new development. The specific episode that prompted his discussion was not the emergence of a new technology per se, but rather a couple's decision to conceive a child in hopes of providing a bone marrow donor for their seriously ill daughter.[17] But it seems a reasonable extension to imagine his criticism being applied to the way many bioethicists react to new technological innovations—the moral rule that a wag once labeled, "Never do anything for the first time."

The field of bioethics looks very different to John Evans. He liked the bioethics business much better in the good old days when those with primarily theological training dominated the field. Since the secular crowd took over, Evans believes that bioethics has degenerated into a cheering section for any new technology that might come along.[18] What seems most interesting about any implied debate between Evans and Rachels about how bioethics responds to technological innovation is the sense that each feels like a member of a beleaguered minority—that whatever position he personally favors, the bulk of bioethicists disagrees with.

Since I know of no scientific survey of bioethicists on what we all think of new technologies, let us turn away from this hypothetical debate and ask what we *should* think. A starting point might be a line of argument that Evans would presumably favor and that Rachels would reject out of hand—Leon Kass's famous essay on human reproductive cloning, in which he appeared to embrace irrationalism as an ethical method.[19] If we cannot think of any good reasons to oppose human cloning, and yet sense a visceral repugnance to the idea, we should go with our gut, as some would say, rather than allow the lack of knock-down rational arguments to deter us. What is going on here? Did Kass simply lose it?[20] Or did he call us to a higher standard for bioethics?

I think several things are going on; but I wish to focus on only one of them. I take Kass in this essay to be situating his specific argument against cloning within a larger tradition of argument, one that Evans attributes more to the theologically than to the philosophically inclined ethicist. This tradition has most often been trotted out, within bioethics, when the technology of concern deals with human reproduction, but there is no reason why only reproductive technologies are relevant to the argument. The argument goes: Many if not most new technologies have two sets of effects. One set is the intended effects, which are often viewed as benefits—such as, in the case of IVF, the ability of childless couples to have children of "their own."[21] The potential benefits are stressed by the scientists who develop and then promote the new technology, are easy to understand, and often sound very compelling. This creates an initial sense of an ethical imperative to implement the technology.

The second set of effects is harder to discern. This set includes subtle changes that may arise in social relationships and ultimately in our own basic sense of who we are as human beings. These effects, while subtle, can ultimately be much longer-lasting and farther-reaching than the new technology itself. Moreover, once unleashed upon the world, the genie represented by this second set of effects can hardly ever be put back into the bottle. The mythical image of the opening of Pandora's box seems to capture with a vengeance what is feared here. The challenge is for serious thinkers about medicine and biomedical science—bioethicists—to discern these more subtle effects and call out appropriate warnings in time.

There are two reasons why one might simply dismiss this line of argument. First, it is clearly a "conservative" type of argument, in the classical and etymological sense of this now-often-misapplied word. It signals a degree of comfort with the past and distrust of the future. An important part of what is wrong with a new technology, according to this argument, is that it is new. If one happens not to be this sort of conservative in one's general approach and viewpoint, such an argument will seem distinctly uncongenial.

The other reason to dismiss this argument out of hand is that it has an irritating *ad hominem* quality. The defenders of the new technology assess the risks and benefits of the procedure, and offer reasons to believe that the benefits will be substantial and the risks minimal. The Kass-Evans crowd replies, "Well, that's what you think, because you have focused only on the obvious, superficial aspects of the technology. We more careful reasoners have looked deeper and have seen things that ought to worry any thoughtful student of the human condition." The defenders retort, "What, exactly, is worrying you? We have read your arguments carefully and have tried to identify the specific concerns that you have, so that we could offer empirical facts that might address those concerns. But all we find in the end is smoke and mirrors." And the conservatives come back with, "Well, of course it seems to you like a lot of smoke and mirrors. But that again simply shows how subtle and discerning we are, and how crude and superficial you are (just what one would expect from a bunch of utilitarians, in fact)."

From the "liberal's" point of view, every attempt to move the argument in the direction of a reasonable debate over the pros and cons of the new technology is met with this smug assertion of both intellectual and moral superiority. Kass seems to be claiming in his essay on cloning that even if he cannot provide compelling reasons, his gut tells him that cloning is distasteful, and his gut is such a finely tuned instrument of moral discernment that we ought to trust what it says implicitly. This way of discussing the issues (or rather avoiding discussion) is exasperating to say the least.[22] More philosophically, it seems to be a claim that the arguments against the technology are non-falsifiable, and therefore in one sense empirically meaningless.

The problems raised by the Kass-Evans mode of argument may explain a phenomenon commented on by historian and bioethics critic M.L. Tina Stevens. Stevens chides bioethicists for their role in the California referendum, Proposition 71, to provide state support for embryonic stem cell research. Stevens is most outraged by the way that scientist-advocates for the proposition overhyped the medical results of stem cell research, promising therapeutic breakthroughs both much faster, and with much greater certainty, than any sober assessment of the record of this line of research to date would justify.[23] She argues that bioethicists in particular should have rushed into print to condemn these falsehoods, and that the field largely failed in its responsibility to do so.[24] I agree fully that the posturing by the defenders of stem cell research was irresponsible, yet I also sympathize to some degree with the bioethicists who hesitated publicly to condemn them. The public is likely to classify people and arguments on the simplistic basis of being "for" or "against" a public issue. Bioethicists who opposed stem cell research because it was overhyped might well have been reluctant to allow anyone to think that they had joined the crowd that opposes stem cell research because it is a form of cloning, and who asserts that cloning is immoral because one simply knows in one's gut that it causes a cheapening of human life.

## :: Reasons for Bioethics to Be Skeptical about Technology

Having now given two reasons why one might have no patience at all with the conservative argument, let me try to defend that mode of argument to a certain extent. Despite its irritating qualities, the argument might some of the time at least prove valid.

At one level, the argument calls attention to a basic feature of our humanity. We humans (indeed, we apes) are by nature tool-makers and tool-users. Our tools can have a major impact on the world that we inhabit. Included within that impact is the reflexive impact that the use of the tool can have on ourselves and how we view ourselves. Once we have deployed certain types of tools, we are no longer able to see ourselves as *not* using such tools. In past centuries, we began to use clocks and optical instruments as ways of observing and measuring the world, and as a result came to see ourselves and our knowledge in a new way. In the present era the same is true of our use of computers. It has become harder and harder *not* to see ourselves as in some sense the extension of the computer, and not to see the human brain as a sort of computer.

It is very unlikely that these alterations in humanity's view of itself were ever a consciously considered part of the list of pros and cons that preceded the adoption of any of these technologies when they were first introduced. And yet the total eventual impact on who we are and what manner of world we inhabit has been, and is, vast. If another example is needed, think of all the changes in American society and thought brought about by the introduction and widespread use of the automobile.

I have noted how hard it is to think, in advance, of the subtle and yet extensive ways in which a new technology may alter our perceptions of our being. Does the *difficulty* in thinking of these effects constitute a reason *not to try to think* about these effects? If thinking clearly in advance about these effects is difficult, but not impossible, why should it *not* be a part of the task of bioethics in confronting new technologies?

It may seem that up to this point I have been dismissive of aspects of the bioethics enterprise that have their roots in theology and religion. So it is time to recall some of the observations made in the earlier chapter on bioethics' interdisciplinary base. In discussing the role of religion in bioethics, we saw how David Barnard called upon the physician to emulate the priest's "prophetic" voice. He specifically praised the prophetic voice of medicine as it might be raised against two "idolatries"— the idolatry of technology and the idolatry of the marketplace (which are often closely linked).[25] What Barnard here calls upon medicine to perform would seem even more clearly to be a task of bioethics.

There is a final reason for bioethics to respond skeptically to the emergence of new technologies. According to this reason, this might be a two-level skepticism. First, bioethicists might be skeptical about the technology itself. More important, bioethicists should be skeptical about their own level of interest in and fascination with the technology, and new technologies generally. This is because the fascination with new technologies reveals a class bias within the field. These new technologies are, for the most part (to be as blunt and unkind about it as possible), the toys of the world's wealthy upper crust. Solomon Benatar, Abdallah Daar, and Peter Singer recently felt it necessary to remind us that in 1994, 45 percent of the world's population had to get by on 4 percent of the world's gross domestic product. At the same time, the top 385 billionaires in the world had a combined personal wealth equal to 4 percent of total GDP.[26] If we wonder which of those two groups might expect to reap the benefits of cutting-edge biomedical technologies, it is unlikely to be the world's poorest 45 percent.

A vague sense of the unseemliness of bioethics' near-exclusive focus on new technologies, at the same time (as we saw in the previous chapter) that issues of global public health and global social justice are marginalized, is increasingly being voiced by those in our field who would prick our conscience.[27] This conscience-pricking must be done with careful regard for the distinction between bioethicists individually and collectively. Any individual member of the field might have excellent reasons for electing to focus her research interests on emerging biomedical technologies, and it does not follow at all from such a research focus that she is personally indifferent to the plight of the world's less-well-off citizens. Yet when the field as a whole seems to pay such disproportionate attention to these technologies, then some sort of explanation is called for.

It is also indicative of the state of the bioethics "culture wars" that this complaint, about a fascination with new technologies being linked with a neglect for basic issues in global justice, seems not to emanate from the so-called conservative wing of the bioethics establishment, despite that group's purportedly anti-technology bias. At the risk of caricature, one might accuse the conservative bioethicists of dividing technologies into two categories. One type is evil because it messes with God's "natural" plan for human beings. One might make money off such technology in a capitalist society, but it would still be wrong. The other sort of technology is neutral with respect to God and "human nature"; it simply reflects the fact that God gave humans dominion over the natural world so that they could improve it in accord with their reason and will. This second sort of technology is fair game for capitalist profits. If the world's poor do not have enough money to purchase these latter technologies, it simply shows that they have not worked hard enough and so do not deserve the privilege. The same God that created the natural world also created markets; and if you end up on the short end in the global market economy, well, that is simply God's will.[28] Eric Cohen, then editor of *The New Atlantis*, a self-proclaimed conservative bioethics journal, very responsibly took his fellow conservatives to task for being insufficiently concerned about justice for the poor.[29]

I will return soon to the question of what sorts of technological issues might concern bioethicists if we took concerns about global justice more seriously. First, let us be sure that power is on the table for discussion.


## ⠶ Power and New Technologies

Clare Williams, of King's College, London, conducted interviews with the staff of two hospital maternal-fetal units in that city. These units perform procedures including diagnoses of congenital defects and fetal surgery to correct defects such as diaphragmatic hernia.[30]

In arguing that the ethical dilemmas faced by the staff she interviewed are truly "unprecedented," Williams lists the following characteristics:

> ...the uniqueness of the maternal-fetal relationship; decision making based on what is often risk and probability-based information; the option of obtaining a definitive diagnosis [through an intervention such as amniocentesis] which may itself result in miscarriage; the influence of enhanced visualization technologies; decision making in a highly-charged moral area, where both partners may have differing views about available options; the rhetorical emphasis within prenatal screening of non-directive, value-free counselling and informed choice. Obviously there are wider influences on such decisions, including prevailing social values and the cultural meaning of, for example, disability.[31]

One could quibble with the "unprecedented" claim. For example, many years ago, Al Jonsen identified the peculiar ethical difficulties of decisions in the neonatal intensive care unit with the fact that almost all prognostic information available about very-low-birthweight infants was statistical and probabilistic.[32] The impossibility of truly value-free and non-directive genetic counseling has been admitted by bioethicists and practitioners in that field.[33]

One could also quibble, perhaps more forcefully, with the claim that the relationship that shapes the peculiar ethical dilemmas in these units is the *maternal–fetal* relationship. It is worth noting that Williams does not claim that the new technologies have *altered* an existing relationship between mother and fetus; it is quite consistent with her hypotheses that the ethically problematic features of that relationship antedated any of these technological developments.[34] Nevertheless it seems problematic that the interview materials that Williams cites can be interpreted in quite a different way. She quotes a midwife, "everyone is so preoccupied with what's OK for the fetus that we actually forget what the mother has to go through...consideration is given to the mother, but not to the same extent and maybe that's not a good thing."[35] This quote in particular seems to suggest that what the new technology has changed is the relationship between the staff and the mother, not between the mother and the fetus.[36] As this same midwife points out, "we call it the Fetal Medicine Unit, but in fact that's not true because you actually have to go through the mother in order to get to the fetus..."[37]

Bioethics has previously addressed issues like court-ordered Caesarian sections and the surreptitious testing of pregnant women for illicit drug use.[38] The power implications of those activities seemed clear. Medical staff, abetted by the legal system, were exercising power over the bodies of pregnant women, and claiming justification for this use of power by virtue of assuming the role of advocates for the health of the fetus. Most women who end up in the maternal-fetal units where Williams did her research came, by contrast, voluntarily, and were eager to comply with the staff's recommendations. The women's voluntary compliance might therefore have obscured the fact that the same general sort of power was being wielded. Maternal-fetal specialists assume a moral authority because they are supposedly dedicated to furthering the interests of the fetus; the "good" pregnant mother-to-be is one who acts responsibly for the protection of her fetus's health. This creates a setting in which the woman may be reluctant to refuse any technological intervention offered, even if it is highly invasive and unlikely to work.

What, exactly, is the relationship between these new technologies and the perceived social pressure on the pregnant woman to accept these interventions? Here, Williams is less helpful than we might like. She admits that often "the technology seemed to have a momentum almost of its own."[39] As further analysis, she proposes:

> So although I am not stating that women are "passive victims" of reproductive technologies, I would argue that women's choices and the roles that they play as active participants in the socialisation of medical

innovation, are made within the context of familial, social, cultural and economic constraints. For example, practitioners can have a powerful ideological impact in "shaping the understanding women have of what their experience of pregnancy should be, and how 'responsible' women should act." As practitioners in this study noted, pregnant women (and practitioners themselves) could feel an imperative to "do something," including undergoing fetal surgery with a low chance of success.[40]

One would wish to know more, even granting that we have here a complex web of social causes linked by bidirectional arrows. What role is played by the development of *specific* new fetal technologies, as opposed to a *general* faith in our society that we can turn to technology to solve problems, and that a person who refuses to utilize these technologies is "not really trying hard enough"? What are the respective roles played by the woman's own desires for a healthy baby, social and cultural expectations for how a "responsible" mother should behave, and the "powerful ideological impact" of the physician?

Williams looks at a certain set of novel technologies from the vantage point of a highly developed society in which a national health service bears (I assume) most of the financial costs, and so sees a set of issues involving individual choice. By contrast, "today's biological technologies" look quite different to Pushpa M. Bhargava, striving to address them from "an Indian point of view."[41] Bhargava is well aware of technologies that affect human reproduction. But he pays considerably more attention to technologies that affect food crops and seed production, especially genetically modified foods—topics that have generated little interest or concern among U.S. bioethicists. Instead of questions of individual choice, he often finds instances of the exploitation of developing countries and their citizens by large international corporations. Sometimes he finds his own government working diligently to protect the interests of its citizens; sometimes he finds the government, apparently with its eyes on the short-term rupees, making common cause with the corporations to the detriment of Indian interests.

Bhargava finds the most pressing ethical questions regarding new biotechnology to be the potential for discrimination and exploitation, both within and among nations. His concerns highlight the tendency of American bioethicists to look upon new technologies *as technologies*, and perhaps to be slow to appreciate that they are at the same time commercial enterprises. His comments remind us how slow American bioethics has been to appreciate the problems posed by the concentration of economic power in the hands of large pharmaceutical companies, and how this has altered the very fabric of medical research and medical education.[42]

## :: A Developing-World Case Study: Clean Water in Benin

Closer to Bhargava's account of the ethical issues raised from the Indian point of view than to Williams's investigation of maternal-fetal technology in London is a case study of a "sustainable" water and sanitation project for the village of Azové in coastal Benin in West Africa. The village became the focus of a student learning project designed by Bradley Striebig and his colleagues in the Department of Civil Engineering, Gonzaga University.[43]

The life expectancy in Benin is fifty-one years, comparing favorably to a number of other African nations (especially those with serious AIDS epidemics) where the life expectancy is closer to forty years. It is estimated that, in rural areas of Benin, 36 percent of the population has access to clean water and 14 percent to adequate sanitary facilities. The Gonzaga team focused their attention on a school in Azové which currently is served by a one-inch water pipe with a hose faucet, dispensing water from a shallow well via gravity flow. The water tested positive for coliform bacteria and other pathogens. Students from the school currently go outdoors to relieve themselves in the fields; the village has two latrines considered to be of poor design that are little used. Approximately half the children under 16 are affected by cholera (which is not recognized by the local people to be a water-borne infection), and half of the entire village is affected by malaria; a significant but unknown number have AIDS. There is a small local health clinic that the locals are reluctant to use for reasons the authors were unable to discover.

Against this background, the Gonzaga engineering students considered investing $10,000 in a sustainable clean-water supply and sanitation program. The characteristics of the technology investigated included its use of local materials and local labor, contributing to the local economy, and the ability of the community to maintain the facility without large infusions of new money in the future and with existing levels of skill and education. The authors did not describe in detail the water facility they contemplated building. They stated that toilet facilities for all residents of the village were not a part of their own project. They did, however, believe that with appropriate training, local businesses could manufacture composting toilets for Azové and sur-rounding communities at an affordable cost. They imagined that the water filtering system they proposed would reduce the number of coli-form bacteria by 99 percent, and the composting toilet system would reduce the load of these bacteria by 90 percent.

The specific ethical problem the students then addressed was the tension between short-term and long-term relief efforts. Initially it seemed absurd to the students that one would spend $10,000 on a water facility that would take years to demonstrate results, when the health problems of the community were so pressing and when the same money could be invested in so many ways that would produce more immediate results. The authors considered only one alternative investment, immu-nizations. They calculated that in the first year, the water-sanitation plan would cost $713 per life saved while an immunization program could save a life for $175. By five years out, however, the cost per life saved began to favor the water program. The immunization program would continue to require a new infusion of the same funds annually while the water system was, in theory, sustainable without very much ongoing expenditure (that is, the authors anticipated maintenance costs as only 10 percent of total costs). The Gonzaga faculty and students con-cluded that spending the money on the water and sanitation system was ethically defensible.

It might seem that this ethics exercise was artificially constructed, and that the answer is clear from the outset. Everyone knows that clean drinking water is a very basic public health need in developing countries and can save many more lives, at much lower cost, than ini-tially investing more in medical care. Everyone knows that economic sustainability is a good thing in planning such projects. So how could there even be a debate about the appropriateness of this expenditure of $10,000?

I must, however, bear in mind that I write these words within a warm, snug house with a full stomach. If I were in the village of Azové, face to face with the people who have to bear the burden of disease, poverty, and limited life opportunities, I might feel much more acutely the moral imperative to do something *now* to alter their plight. My con-frontation with the immediacy of their neediness would, according to the ethical teachings of Levinas, be a much more human, moral, and generally satisfactory response than engaging in cost-benefit analyses.

My suspicions of the water system might be magnified after reading some of Paul Farmer's polemical writings on bioethics and international health, in which he regards "sustainable" as one of the buzzwords indicative of a neoliberal approach to development. If I grasp his meaning, "sustainability" usually refers to the likelihood that an intervention can be maintained with the use solely of local resources. In turn, it takes the local structure as a given. That local structure, Farmer points out, often consists of a wealthy elite that makes common cause with global corporations to create a form of "development" that enriches the elite and the corporations, while keeping the poor mired in poverty. What social justice demands is not something "sustainable" in the face of this structure of exploitation and violence, but the willingness to declare that that structure is itself unsustainable.[44] It may be that in the Benin case, the definition and criteria for sustainability are more benign. The mere fact that the word has been invoked should not, however, put an end to ethical inquiry.

Finally, I would be concerned about the appropriateness of this solution for the people of Azové because the account by the Gonzaga professors is very scanty in supplying any evidence that the options have been explained to them and that the water system is the one that they favor. Reading between the lines, one sees commendable examples of having consulted with the local community—at least with the administrators of the school, at any rate. The authors know that the latrines that now exist are considered inadequate, and that if the new water and sanitation system were implemented, the school administrators plan to next build a nursing station to provide additional health services. The overall design of the water and sanitation system appear to have been endorsed by the Songhai Center in Porto-Novo, Benin, a respected non-governmental organization addressing local needs.

On the other hand, there is no direct report of any consultation with the community regarding the possible uses of $10,000; and it seems somewhat worrisome that the authors are unclear as to why the locals do not want to use the existing health center. One would have imagined that adequate dialogue with the community about how they perceived their health needs would have answered that question. In the final analysis, one has to wonder about the "sustainability" of a project that is plunked down in an African village without a sense of ownership by the local people, simply because a group of experts in Spokane think that it is cost-effective.

In sum, I have considered an ethical problem relating to a new technology, and noted a number of questions related to one proposed solution. The discussion has gone in a rather different direction than most bioethical analyses of new technologies. If this discussion seems atypical, it may be that our fixation on problems of technologies as they arise in the developed world has distorted our vision, and that we need to attend much more broadly to all bioethical questions related to new technologies in various global environments.

NOTES TO CHAPTER 11

1. The so-called "Georgetown mantra," named after the university that houses the Kennedy Institute of Ethics, is a wag's way of referring to the famous four principles of Beauchamp and Childress's *Principles of Biomedical Ethics* (autonomy, non-maleficence, beneficence, justice). In referring to my mantra tongue-in-cheek as the "Hastings" mantra I don't intend to suggest that the scholars at the Hastings Center in Garrison, New York, today are still under its throes, any more than I would suggest that all members of today's Kennedy Institute slavishly worship at the principlist altar.

2. "Recent advances in biology and medicine make it increasingly clear that we are rapidly acquiring greater powers to modify and perhaps control the capacities and activities of men by direct intervention into and manipulation of their bodies and minds.... All of these developments raise profound and difficult questions of theory and practice...[W]e can ill afford to wait until the crush of events forces us to make hasty and often ill-considered decisions." Mondale WF. The issues before us. *Hastings Cent Rep* 1(1), June 1971; "Today, however, extraordinary advances in the biological and medical sciences are raising new and serious ethical, social, and legal problems, not only for physicians, but for society in general." Complex problems for MDs: as science gains, moral dilemmas intensify. *Am Med News*, May 1, 1972: 7; "Remarkable advances were being made in organ transplantation, human experimentation, prenatal diagnosis of genetic disease, prolongation of life and control of human behavior—and each advance posed specific problems requiring that scientific knowledge be matched with ethical insight." Institute of Society, Ethics and the Life Sciences. *Hastings Cent Studies* 1(1), 1973: inside front cover.

3. Litton P. Nanoethics: what's new? *Hastings Cent Rep* 37(1):22–25, 2007.

4. My account here is taken from Vinten-Johansen P, Brody H, Paneth N, et al. *Cholera, chloroform, and the science of medicine: A life of John Snow.* New York: Oxford University Press, 2003, pp. 185–98.

5. Jeremy Greene takes this understanding to the next level in his history of pharmacotherapeutics for chronic disease in the later part of the twentieth century. He demonstrates that the development of a new mode of treating a disease may reflexively alter our understanding of the nature of the disease itself; Greene JA. *Prescribing by numbers: drugs and the definition of disease.* Baltimore: Johns Hopkins University Press, 2007.

6. Stanley Reiser has sketched out the steps needed to turn the existing thermometers of the day into an instrument that was the right size and

shape to register the patient's temperature, and that could then retain that information accurately long enough for it to be noted and recorded; Reiser SJ. *Medicine and the reign of technology*. New York: Cambridge University Press, 1978, pp. 110–21.

7. Consider, for example, a description of typhoid fever from 1847: "Following the chill or rigor,...there is, almost always, increased heat of the skin. In many patients, it is quite moderate in degree and pretty uniformly diffused over the body. In others, the morbid heat is high and burning, and not unfrequently very unequally distributed....This morbid heat...is subject to certain variations in the course of each day...more commonly there are two [increases in heat] each day. In the early period of the disease, the most strongly marked exacerbation is usually in the afternoon....The state of the skin, in regard to dryness and moisture, is quite different in different patients..."; Bartlett E. *The history, diagnosis, and treatment of the fevers of the United States*. Philadelphia: Lea and Blanchard, 1847, pp. 41–42.

8. On the progression from purely narrative descriptions of cases in charts in U.S. hospitals to the inclusion of quantitative data such as pulse, respiration, temperature, and blood pressure, and some of the implications for therapeutics, see Warner JH. *The therapeutic perspective: medical practice, knowledge, and identity in America, 1820–1885*. Cambridge, MA: Harvard University Press, 1986, pp. 153–9.

9. I have been unable to relocate my original source for the discussion of the way that the advent of the recording clinical thermometer altered the respective roles of the physician and nurse. I am grateful to Jason Glenn and Dayle DeLancey for reassurances that my summary here appears to be historically plausible.

10. Howell JD. *Technology and the hospital: transforming patient care in the early twentieth century*. Baltimore: Johns Hopkins University Press, 1995.

11. Warner notes that when the first fever/temperature charts or curves appeared in U.S. hospital records, they were hand-drawn by house physicians on the pages intended for handwritten narrative notes. A few years later, graphic representations of temperature curves appear on preprinted forms, but these had to be pasted onto the pages. Warner JH. *The therapeutic perspective: medical practice, knowledge, and identity in America, 1820–1885*, pp. 153–9. Howell takes this story forward to note that by 1925, these preprinted and standardized forms had become much more common and also much more efficiently designed, making their insertion into the medical record much simpler; indeed the record now contained more such forms than it did narrative; Howell JD. *Technology and the hospital: transforming patient care in the early twentieth century*. Baltimore: Johns Hopkins University Press, 1995, pp. 42–56.

12. Kass LR. Babies by means of in vitro fertilization: unethical experiments on the unborn? *N Engl J Med* 285:1174–9, 1971; Ramsey P. Shall we "reproduce"? I. The medical ethics of in vitro fertilization. *JAMA* 220:1346–50, 1972; Ramsey P. Shall we "reproduce"? II. Rejoinders and future forecast. *JAMA* 220:1480–5, 1972.

13. Ramsey P. Shall we "reproduce"? II. Rejoinders and future forecast, 1480–85.
14. Brody H. Genetic engineering: sizing up the arguments in the post–Louise Brown era. In: Teichler-Zallen D, Clements CD (eds.). *Science and morality*. Lexington, MA: Lexington Books, 1982, pp. 139–53; Brody H. Ethics, technology, and the human genome project. *J Clin Ethics* 2:278–81, 1991.
15. Murray TH. Even if it worked, cloning wouldn't bring her back. *Washington Post*, April 8, 2001:B1.
16. Rachels J. When philosophers shoot from the hip: a report from America. *Bioethics* 5:67–71, 1991.
17. Rachels J. When philosophers shoot from the hip: a report from America.
18. Evans JH. *Playing God? Human genetic engineering and the rationalization of public bioethical debate*. Chicago: University of Chicago Press, 2002. Evans must have been disappointed with the example set by Joseph Fletcher, in many ways the major pioneer of the new medical ethics in the 1950s, a professor of religious ethics who appears never to have met a new technology that he didn't like. See, for instance, Fletcher J. *The ethics of genetic control: ending reproductive roulette*. Garden City, NY: Anchor, 1974. In the end, Evans seems sympathetic with the dismissal of Fletcher as a "theologian-turned-technocrat" who had turned into an apologist for the scientists' point of view: Evans, *Playing God*, pp. 63–7.
19. Kass L. The wisdom of repugnance. *New Republic* 216 (June 2, 1997):17–26.
20. It appears that Kass gained it rather than lost it, as this essay may have been the single most important reason why he was appointed the chair of the President's Council on Bioethics under the Bush Administration. A cynic might claim that the essay was written more for its political than for its intellectual effectiveness.
21. This part of the argument, incidentally, illustrates why one may oppose human reproductive cloning on very solid grounds without accepting any of Kass's considerations. The benefits of human reproductive cloning ought to be weighed against its risks. I have yet to learn any substantial *benefit* that will result from human reproductive cloning that could not much more easily be achieved in some much simpler fashion in the vast majority of cases; most of the purported "benefits" result from simple, factual misunderstandings about cloning (e.g., that I could clone an individual using my DNA and then use that body as a source of organs for transplant, as if the cloned individual would not be a human being with full legal rights under law). Given the lack of any realistic benefit, all it would take would be a small risk of harm to negate any ethical defense of cloning.
22. The sense of exasperation is increased when the assertions of smug moral superiority emanate from a group whose greatest pleasure in life sometimes appears to be in dictating to the rest of us how we ought or ought not to have sex and reproduce.
23. Stevens MLT. Intellectual capital and voting booth bioethics: a contemporary historical critique. In: Eckenwiler LA, Cohn FG (eds.).

*The ethics of bioethics: mapping the moral landscape.* Baltimore: Johns Hopkins University Press, 2007, pp. 59–73.

24. The one exception that Stevens admits, an op-ed column by Daniel Callahan, actually provides quite a good example of the sort of argument that Stevens wishes more bioethicists had made: Callahan D. Combining hope, hype and hucksterism. *San Diego Union-Tribune,* October 22, 2004, http://www.signonsandiego.com/uniontrib/20041022/news_z1e22callaha.html (accessed November 11, 2007). Callahan, who has made a long career of expressing his skepticism about the human value of new medical technologies, skewers the hype promulgated by the stem-cell defenders while refusing to adopt the religious and ethical presumptions of the Kass-Evans contingent.

25. Barnard D. The physician as priest, revisited. *J Religion Health* 24:272–86, 1985; p. 284; see Chapter 2 for a more extended discussion.

26. Benatar SR, Daar AS, Singer PA. Global health ethics: the rationale for mutual caring. *International Affairs* 79:107–38, 2003; see table on p. 113.

27. See, for instance, Turner L. Bioethics in a multicultural world: medicine and morality in pluralistic settings. *Health Care Analy* 11:99–117, 2003; Marshall P, Koenig B. Accounting for culture in a globalized bioethics. *J Law Med Ethics* 32:252–66, 2004; Farmer P, Campos NG. New malaise: bioethics and human rights in the global era. *J Law Med Ethics* 32:243–51, 2004; Zoloth L. I want you: notes toward a theory of hospitality. In: Eckenwiler LA, Cohn FG, eds. *The ethics of bioethics: mapping the moral landscape.* Baltimore: Johns Hopkins University Press, 2007, pp. 205–19.

28. A brief summary of the relationship between neoclassical market economics and religious evangelism, going back to the nineteenth century and the British government's response to the Irish potato famine, is found in Bigelow G. Let there be markets: the evangelical roots of economics. *Harper's Magazine* 310(1860, May 2005):33–8.

29. Cohen E. Conservative bioethics and the search for wisdom. *Hastings Cent Rep* 36(1):44–56, 2006.

30. Williams C. Dilemmas in fetal medicine: premature applications of technology or responding to women's choice? *Sociology Health Illn* 28:1–20, 2006.

31. Williams C. Dilemmas in fetal medicine: premature applications of technology or responding to women's choice?; quote on p. 8.

32. Jonsen AR. Ethics, the law, and the treatment of seriously ill newborns. In: Doudera AE, Peters JD (eds.) *Legal and ethical aspects of treating critically and terminally ill patients.* Ann Arbor, MI: AUPHA Press, 1982, pp. 236–41.

33. See, for example, Ehrich K, Williams C, Farsides B, et al. Choosing embryos: ethical complexity and relational autonomy in staff accounts of PGD. *Sociol Health Illn* 29:1091–106, 2007.

34. On the other hand, causative force might be attributed to the imaging technologies that allow the parents to *see* the fetus today in ways previously impossible, and thereby (many argue) alter the relationship.

35. Williams C. Dilemmas in fetal medicine: premature applications of technology or responding to women's choice?; quote on p. 6.

36. I am grateful to Judy Andre for pointing out on a number of occasions that what the bioethics literature commonly refers to as "maternal-fetal conflict" almost always is, in reality, maternal-physician conflict.

37. Williams C. Dilemmas in fetal medicine: premature applications of technology or responding to women's choice?; quote on p. 6.

38. Board of Trustees, American Medical Association. Legal interventions during pregnancy: court-ordered medical treatments and legal penalties for potentially harmful behavior by pregnant women. *JAMA* 264:2663–70, 1990; Annas GJ. Testing poor pregnant women for cocaine–physicians as police investigators. *N Engl J Med* 344:1729–32, 2001.

39. Williams C. Dilemmas in fetal medicine: premature applications of technology or responding to women's choice?; quote on p. 9. This observation leads Williams to repeat a part of the Hastings mantra, "One key aim is to encourage more widespread debate about the potential dilemmas which may arise from [new technologies], before, rather than following their introduction" (quote on p. 17).

40. Williams C. Dilemmas in fetal medicine: premature applications of technology or responding to women's choice?; quote on p. 16, citations omitted.

41. Bhargava PM. The social, moral, ethical, legal, and political implications of today's biological technologies: an Indian point of view. *Biotechnol J* 1:34–46, 2006.

42. Kassirer JP. *On the take: how medicine's complicity with big business can endanger your health.* New York: Oxford University Press, 2005; Brody H. *Hooked: ethics, the medical profession, and the pharmaceutical industry.* Lanham, MD: Rowman and Littlefield, 2007; Elliott C. Pharma goes to the laundry: public relations and the business of medical education. *Hastings Cent Rep* 34(5):18–23, 2004

43. Striebig BA, Jantzen T, Rowden K. Ethical considerations of the short-term and long-term health impacts, costs, and educational value of sustainable development projects. *Sci Eng Ethics* 12:345–54, 2006.

44. Farmer P. *Pathologies of power: health, human rights, and the new war on the poor.* Berkeley: University of California Press, 2003; see, for example, p. 156 and p. 226.

# 12 ::

# Conclusion

Here I want to address two different tasks. First, some additional topics belong, in my opinion, on the "future" list, and yet for various reasons did not lend themselves to chapter-length expansion. I want now to list briefly some of those additional topics.

Second, I have been arguing all along for a bioethics that attends more carefully to disparities in power. I do this not merely so that we can be intellectually stimulated—even though we have seen all along how interesting theoretical developments follow as a result of the new focus I suggest. I propose that we should, as a general rule, do more to speak up on behalf of those who lack power, especially when we can find ways to assist them to speak for themselves. This in turn suggests, as we move from theory to practice, that bioethics ought to adopt a more activist sense of its mission. I will conclude the volume by discussing what such an activist bioethics might entail.

## :: Other "Future" Topics

Recall from Chapter 1 what criteria are used to designate a topic that belongs on our list. First, the topic must currently be receiving less attention from mainstream bioethics than it seems to warrant. Second, addressing the topic will move bioethics away from Kuhnian "normal" thinking and enhance the possibility of real intellectual advance.

Using these criteria, one could have recommended that all of the following topics be included in this volume.

*Professionalism in medicine and health care.* I elected not to include a chapter on professionalism because it seemed to risk undermining a central theme of this book. Professionals, by definition, wield a good deal of power. A bioethics that focuses especially on professionalism, particularly in medicine, risks identification with the powerful and the possible neglect of the concerns of those lacking power. Professionalism also might seem a poor subject for inclusion on our list because a great deal has been written about it in the past decade—even though much of the writing does not come from bioethicists.

Despite these concerns, I think both that professionalism needs bioethical attention, and also that careful thinking about professionalism may move bioethics in useful directions.[1] First, despite the volume of ink spilled so far, the precise definition of "professionalism" has not been settled, and to some degree various authors are talking past each other as a result. To a large degree, the sizeable literature on professionalism has been generated by medical educators, and there is a felt need to develop curriculum and most especially, evaluation strategies.[2] One may worry that we are rushing to teach professionalism, and to evaluate how successful our teaching has been, before we are quite sure what it is.[3] Understanding better what professionalism is would also entail better understanding its historical evolution.[4]

Addressing professionalism forthrightly as a central issue in bioethics would bring about two valuable developments. First, it would probably be found that a full explication of professionalism will require a virtue-ethics approach, and virtue ethics remains somewhat underrepresented in today's bioethics armamentarium. Second, understanding professionalism would also cause us to take very seriously the need to address forthrightly the concept that is often seen as opposed to professionalism: self-interest. The physician's legitimate, ethically important self-interest is typically glossed over or simply ignored in the rush to celebrate professionalism, which dooms "professionalism" to degenerate into empty rhetoric. Yet the number of bioethics studies that look seriously at physician self-interest is quite small.[5]

*Business ethics in health care.* As we saw when we discussed pay-for-performance in Chapter 4, professionalism is often contrasted with commercial or business behavior. That presupposes that we know what ethical rules business behavior follows. Many physicians imagine that "business ethics" is an oxymoron. Presumably, bioethicists have studied ethics, and therefore are aware that there exists a field known as business ethics; but few have gone into much depth in becoming acquainted with that field.

Since large institutions are involved with health care, and since those institutions must be run as businesses, it would seem to be valuable to create more "cross-talk" (as we discussed in Chapter 2) between bioethics and business ethics. Such cross-talk might reveal that there is more common ground than was initially thought, and that business ethics demands more restraint and social responsibility than many of us had imagined.[6] For example, Leonard Weber has argued that if pharmaceutical companies followed optimally ethical business practices, major reforms would occur, in a direction that was quite favorable toward enhanced medical professionalism.[7]

*Aging and dementia.* I admit to skepticism about whether new discoveries in neuroscience rise to the level of justifying an entire new sub-field within bioethics called "neuroethics," as many today are advocating. I would have been tempted to list "neuroethics" among the "usual suspects" in Chapter 1 that did not deserve inclusion on the "future" list, except for the fact that neuroethics, broadly understood, would include dementia.[8]

Aging and dementia can be viewed as falling under the general heading of end-of-life care, or alternatively, under disabilities. Neither categorization adequately addresses their unique features. Assuming that aging and dementia equal the "end of life" positions bioethics in the "pro-death" posture that some of its most acerbic critics attribute to it.[9] Using the disabilities lens tends to obscure the fact that almost all of us can expect, if we live long enough, to experience this loss of capabilities and increased dependency.

How are we to understand this phase of dependency and loss of capabilities, within the overall context of a complete human life? The task might seem to be one of correctly placing and understanding certain chapters within the context of one's autobiography. A narrative conception of dementia, in particular, seems on one hand absolutely essential to ethical understanding, and on the other hand extremely elusive. A first-person narrative of dementia, to the extent that it is coherent, invariably signals that the author is only in the very earliest stages of the condition, and so is unable to reflect for us what deepening dementia consists of. Narratives of advanced dementia, by contrast, are almost always the narratives of the caregivers, not of the patient.[10] Those caregiver narratives can in themselves be extremely significant, but they do not answer the deepest ethical questions. Perhaps with more thought and creativity we will find ways to triangulate among different narratives to create a more satisfactory account of the meaning and experience of dementia. This in turn could lead to a much enhanced understanding of how to treat the demented individual with appropriate compassion and dignity.

This completes my own list for "the future of bioethics," though I am sure that with more thought and research I could have added some topics. I now want to address the implicit theme of many of the previous chapters—that I seem to be calling for a greater degree of activism for the field of bioethics on behalf of the less powerful. I will approach the question of activism obliquely by returning to the idea, introduced in Chapter 1, of "bioethics as practice."

## ∷ A Portion of a Bioethicist's Diary

October 11, 2007: I have two lectures to give at the University of California at Irvine, both on ways that the commercial influence of the pharmaceutical industry challenges medical professionalism. This week, a new study was published (which I read on the plane coming in), providing details on the financial involvements of medical school departments with the industry.[11] I have created a blog in order regularly to update the information in my recent book on this topic.[12] Ideally I will find the time in the next day or so to post a new entry on the blog to discuss the recent study. But my wife and I are using the trip to southern California as an opportunity to spend a couple of days with our daughter who lives in San Diego. I am not sure when I can get to the blog.

October 15: My only day in the office this week. I cannot recall how I got myself into this busy of a travel schedule for these few weeks.

October 16: Today's task is to speak about the controversial Texas medical futility statute, at the leadership conference of the Texas Hospital Association. As a newcomer to the state, I finally get to meet some of the key players in the statewide coalition that crafted the original legislation; we agree that we need to become better acquainted. A state legislator discusses the alternative bill that was proposed in the last legislative session. Because I was focusing on the futility discussion, I had forgotten that this bill included a provision that would declare artificial nutrition and hydration to be "ordinary" treatment. The post-Schiavo objections to removing feeding tubes are prompting such legislative efforts around the country. Many of us in bioethics thought this issue had finally been resolved with the Cruzan ruling. Are people not aware of the more recent literature reviews documenting the lack of benefit of tube feeding in the terminally ill and the demented elderly?[13] Maybe our group in Galveston needs to discuss writing a paper for a medical journal to move the issue back to the front burner.

October 17: Now it's off to D.C. for the annual meeting of the American Society for Bioethics and Humanities (ASBH). I get some more reading done on the plane but still have not found the time to update my blog.

October 18: I'm pleased to see that a number of the topics listed in this book are on the ASBH annual meeting program—maybe the future of bioethics will get here before I can finish the book. (When, by the way, will I next have some serious time to work on the manuscript?) I'm looking forward to meeting many old friends and also networking with various colleagues. The program is daunting because so many things are happening at the same time. I had hoped to be able to attend the affinity group meeting on disabilities, given my emerging interest in that area of bioethics, but it looks as if I cannot attend both that meeting and another session I feel that I cannot miss.

October 19: This morning's newspaper has an article about a recent death in Virginia from methicillin-resistant *staphylococcus aureus* (MRSA), also mentioning a recent study that claims that 18,000 deaths annually occur in the U.S. due to this organism.[14] In an odd minute I go online and read the study—it seems as if their statistics are shaky and the estimate of deaths might be inflated. The public will now be scared that a new super-bug is running rampant. I write a weekly health column that appears in two small newspapers. I have columns all set to go for the coming weeks, but maybe I should find time over the weekend to write a new column on the MRSA risk and bump next week's column.

Our Galveston group attending the ASBH meeting has dinner together. I get a few minutes to talk to my bioethicist-gastroenterologist colleague. He agrees with me that perhaps we should write a paper updating the ethical issues around artificial nutrition and hydration. When we all get back I need to call a meeting and see who is interested—and who has time.

October 20: Nancy Scheper-Hughes, a medical anthropologist at UC-Berkeley, presents her work on international organ-trafficking. We had recently had some discussions back in Galveston of the ethics of selling one's organs, but I had no idea things were as bad as this. The descriptions of prominent transplant surgeons consorting with the depths of the criminal underworld to secure a sufficient supply of organs reminds me of Dylan Thomas's screenplay, *The Doctor and the Devils*.[15] Is this an issue we somehow should be doing more to publicize or to protest?

Tod Chambers of Northwestern University is installed as the new president of ASBH. In his address he talks about the division between those who regard the organization as primarily a locus of intellectual exchange and those who believe that they have signed on to a reformist cause, to improve the world. He submits that ASBH can properly serve both goals. His talk is brief and I am not sure that I caught the finer points of his reasoning. I need to see the talk in writing before I can judge whether Tod has given us a genuine blueprint to resolve a long-simmering dispute, or has merely shared some feel-good rhetoric.

By missing the evening session I manage to write the newspaper column on MRSA and e-mail it to my editors, and to get caught up on my e-mail backlog, but still no time to finish updating the blog.

October 21: One of our promising graduate students successfully presents her originally hour-long paper in the fifteen minutes allotted to paper presenters by ASBH. Then I am off to the airport for the flight back to Houston. I have to wait a while for the plane and so have time to write down this "diary" in the gate area. It is the first work I have done on the book manuscript in several weeks.

Judy Andre has noted the importance of seeing bioethics as a practice rather than as simply a body of knowledge. She also calls for the practice of an "engaged" bioethics.[16] In that spirit I have tried to describe a bit of my own "practice" of bioethics during this ten-day period. It seems eminently fair to ask to what extent I was *engaged*.

Lest I appear to have been unduly boastful, I will note immediately all the ways in which I was *not* engaged. During this period of time I gave four public presentations and met a number of new people. But I made no efforts to go "out into the community" and to engage in dialogue with those who do not normally populate the halls of academe or of hospitals. I spent several days in our nation's capital but did not meet with or lobby any elected or appointed officials; nor did I write letters to any of them on pressing public issues. (The unsuccessful effort to override President Bush's veto of the children's health insurance benefit extension occurred during this time, and certainly would seem to have warranted at least a letter to one's congressional representatives.) I did not picket or demonstrate anywhere. I have no evidence that anything in the world was practically changed by any of the activities described in my "diary."

What is an "engaged" bioethics? Is engagement enough? Is it too much?

## ∷ Bioethics: Engaged or Activist?

Andre introduces her idea of "engaged" bioethics also in relation to a meeting of the ASBH—in her case, in October, 2000. The ASBH has undergone considerable internal debate and dissension around the issue of "taking stands." The current bylaws prohibit the organization from adopting a public stand on substantive issues in bioethics, though an amendment was approved that allows the organization to take a stand on issues related to academic freedom of bioethics and humanities faculty and their own ability to take stands as individuals. As Tod Chambers noted at the 2007 meeting, some members believe that ASBH best maintains its integrity as an organization where all intellectual views are welcomed and openly debated, so that "taking a stand" would signal a premature closure of this debate. Other members believe it morally outrageous that ASBH cannot publicly declare its support even for so widely held a position as requiring informed consent from human research subjects.[17]

In 2000, it seemed to Andre that the organization was in fact farther along the road to resolving these differences than later events proved:

> I believe [ASBH] will find a middle way between activism and "informing the debate," a way more tentative and reflective than a political group can be, but more engaged than a purely scholarly group can be. I believe, in other words, that the organization will find a way to participate in a kind of national moral development about health care, health science, and health policy.[18]

Andre later described her work with some local hospitals to draw attention to problems with nursing morale and eventually to make a case for addressing organizational ethics—issues that that particular hospital administration wished rather to sweep under the rug. That project, she added,

> …helped me to articulate the distinction between activism and an engaged bioethics. At one point, thinking that we should intervene on one side of a dispute, we suddenly recognized that our job was to be a resource and a challenge to both sides. We were not neutral about what should be done, but our purpose was to help others *recognize* it as well as carry it out, and simply adding muscle to one side would not have helped. In other situations, however, taking sides might be appropriate, since we would

never choose a side without making our reasoning clear, and never close off further reflection about our choice.[19]

Andre seems very clear on where she stands with regard to the membership divide that Chambers described. Bioethics, says Andre, "is about making a difference."[20] What, then, does she find wrong with activism? It appears that for her, activism is insufficiently "tentative and reflective"; it amounts to using too much muscle and too little reason in favor of the side that one chooses.

By contrast, Lisa Parker argues that bioethics is properly viewed as an activist enterprise and should indeed embrace that self-image.[21] She begins by noting that when individual bioethicists take positions on substantive issues like physician-assisted suicide or embryonic stem-cell research, they are hardly doing anything worth noticing. Taking such stands is "business as usual" for bioethics. The more noteworthy activity might be to *avoid* taking any such stands—the average bioethicist would find that posture much harder to assume, and his interlocutors might accuse him of disingenuousness if he attempted it. Similarly, one need not stretch a point to encourage bioethicists to theorize, or to engage in procedures that look a great deal like rational democratic deliberation. Parker agrees that both bioethics and democratic deliberation typically seek to neutralize power differentials in society by trying to reach agreement based on rational argument and not on threats or force. All these practices would seem to make bioethics different from activism.

But deliberative democracy can engender its own problems. In some instances at least it may prove fraudulent—or, in Marxist terms, generate a false consciousness. It is often the case that the more powerful within society need not resort to threats or force in order to get their way. Appeals to reason may work for them just as well. They may have obtained a relative monopoly on the authority within society to determine what counts as reasonable or what does not; or on the social resources necessary to be viewed as offering the more reasonable position (such as access to research funding). In such instances, democratic deliberation shifts from being the friend of the powerless to being doubly their enemy. It is their enemy first because it allows itself to be used as a means by which the powerful can exert their will. And it is an enemy, second, because it obscures what is really going on—by pretending that it is all a matter of reasoned argument and consensus, deliberative democracy can cover up the fact that the power differential between the haves and have-nots has been increased rather than erased.

What does bioethics do when faced with this sort of failure of deliberative democracy? At its worst, Parker suggests, bioethics allows itself to be seduced by those in power—in particular, those who represent medicine and science. It is all very well for us to insist that we are "outsiders," and that the bioethics faculty member in the medical school never is granted the stature assumed by the physicians and scientists. The fact is that in many ways we are insiders—the physicians and scientists allow us to serve on the faculty, where we frequently earn more money, sometimes considerably more, than our colleagues in the regular humanities departments, as well as enjoying all the special perks that come from being where the action is. If the cost of being allowed inside is not to be too strident in our criticisms of the practices of our physician and scientist colleagues, many of us are all too happy to pay the price.

What does it actually mean to say that bioethicists can be bought off in this manner? Am I pointing out a substantial, practical concern; or am I simply playing around with some sort of postmodernist critique to prove that I am among the academically fashionable crowd? Let's take a minute to examine a more searching analysis of deliberative democracy and bioethics in action.

## ∷ A Case Study: National Bioethics Commissions and Consensus

The role of public bioethics commissions illustrates the tension between activism and deliberative democracy. Susan Kelly has explored the role of such "public bioethics" from the standpoint of science studies—especially the role played by the search for consensus as the preferred method of these commissions.[22]

Physicians and scientists are in a bind when issues arise regarding policies that affect their work, and significant policymakers or other opinion leaders decide that these policy matters raise *ethical* issues. On one hand, the scientific community itself has defined ethical deliberation as outside its boundaries. On the other, scientists do not want to hand over their fate to the decisions of non-scientists. If things work out the way the scientific community would most prefer, the public bioethics commission takes care of the problem. It will be guaranteed that a number of scientists will be appointed to the commission, and will be seen by their fellow commissioners as legitimate content experts in the field of inquiry. The commission might well recommend in the end that research in this field should go forward with certain safeguards and protections—ideally ones that the scientists will not find unduly onerous. The public bioethics commission has performed, for the scientists, a sort of laundering operation. A scientific opinion that would have been rejected because it appears to be self-serving has now been washed and pressed and reappears in its new guise as a "bioethical consensus."

The "consensus" method shows how the scientists and bioethicists have between them remained in control of the process that is put forth as a form of deliberative democracy. Kelly uses for her prime example the U.S. Human Embryo Research Panel convened by the NIH in 1994. To the dismay of the right-to-life political contingent, no one recognized as having a right-to-life position was named as a member of the panel. The commission determined that in order to reach a rational consensus based on the proper scientific facts, it would need to include and consider "thoughtful" positions. In this instance, it appears that the right-to-life point of view was not considered sufficiently "thoughtful" to earn a place at the table.

Kelly cites Jonathan Moreno's philosophical explorations into the justification for "consensus."[23] Moreno in turn mentions John Rawls's model of overlapping consensus.[24] Rawls imagines that parties to a negotiation might each have a different "comprehensive doctrine," a fully worked out set of religious and/or philosophical views about everything of moral significance in human life. In a pluralistic society it is hopeless to imagine that we could ground any "consensus" on completely shared comprehensive doctrines. Rawls insists, however, that to reach consensus on such basic matters as the political structure of a just society, we do not need these comprehensive doctrines to agree *in toto*, or even in the majority of their beliefs and teachings. Thankfully, all we require is that there be a small domain within each doctrine where relevantly similar beliefs are held in common with believers in all the other doctrines. This overlapping consensus regarding the basic political structure of society might include, for instance, the beliefs that slavery is always and everywhere wrong; that opportunities for advancement in society ought not be distributed solely on the basis of family wealth; and that certain basic rights and liberties ought to be guaranteed by the state and not subjected to a majority vote. Rawls thinks it will be easy to reach agreement on a lean subset of such beliefs even among a set of comprehensive doctrines that disagree among themselves dramatically on other, more controversial moral matters. And he also believes that that lean subset will suffice for his purposes.

Reliance on a philosophical theory like overlapping consensus places a public bioethics commission in an interesting position. The scientist members of the commission were presumably appointed for their expertise. And now it seems as if the bioethicists have a similar claim to expertise that justifies their inclusion—and that further justifies accepting what they claim to be the "consensus" as a true moral warrant for policy formulation. The bioethicist can be viewed as an expert in the logical relationship among the various elements of one's comprehensive doctrine. This understanding of how a comprehensive doctrine is put together, as it were, allows the bioethicist to discern the possibility of an overlapping consensus among seemingly-at-odds comprehensive doctrines, and further to explain what beliefs or elements that overlapping consensus consists of.

The scientists are granted credence as experts on the panel because they have *discovered* facts about the world. In the model we have just described, the bioethicists similarly seem to have *discovered* a set of moral "facts" about the possibility for overlapping consensus. The idea that the consensus is in some sense discovered rather than constructed might seem to provide additional justification for adopting certain policies. Notice how differently things would appear if we were instead to describe the commission as having *negotiated* its consensus. That term might much more accurately capture the process that actually occurred. But no one would imagine that a *negotiated* consensus was a particularly good moral basis for policy formulation—especially if we now add the fact that certain interested groups, such as the right-to-life contingent, were denied a seat at the table.

According to the critical perspective sketched here, the work of bioethicists on this public commission is quite the opposite of an *activist* stance. Put simply, bioethics here endorses and defends business as usual in the scientific community; while most of the time the activist seeks to disrupt business as usual.[25] The activist seeks to call into question the current ways that power is allocated; the bioethics commission appears to have been an unquestioning, nonreflective exercise in the power of expertise.


## ⚏ Bioethics' Activist Tendencies

We left Parker listing all the reasons why bioethics might be tempted to allow itself to be seduced by power. But she insists that those temptations are only part of the story. At our best, the theorizing, reflective part of bioethics comes to the rescue. We catch on to the ways that those with power manipulate deliberative democracy for their own advantage, and we analyze and expose those manipulations. Sometimes, admittedly, too much or the wrong kind of theorizing works against us. Parker offers the example of arguments that there is "really" no such thing as "race" as a medical or biological construct, and how such a position might be used by those who wish to deny that racial-ethnic health disparities represent a serious problem of social justice.[26] Yet bioethics is at least capable of identifying the abuses of power and reason in deliberative democracy, and as such has potential as an activist movement.

Parker attributes much of bioethicists' success at activism to its having listened to its feminist practitioners (and critics):

> Bioethics scholarship has taken up many of the key prescriptions of its feminist theorists: attend to structural inequities; include diverse perspectives, especially those of the less powerful; advocate for the material conditions necessary for autonomous choice to be effective and valuable; and recognize the import of people's dependence and relatedness. Combining activist methods of engaging an audience at an emotional level with activist goals of questioning the dominant discursive frame, we offer counternarratives as well as counterarguments. While we are mindful of the problems of representation and the pitfalls of presuming to speak on behalf of others, we give voice to perspectives of those who lack the standing or strength to present their own stories and advocate for their own interests.[27]

Some might argue that bioethics can never be an activist enterprise so long as it resides within the corridors of power, in the halls of science and medicine. Parker suggests two ways to look at this relationship. One possibility is that bioethics is inevitably corrupted by its location within these institutions. But another is that these institutions themselves are not irretrievably or terminally corrupt, else bioethics in its present form would never have been allowed to take hold there:

> Moreover, to the extent that as bioethicists we have power or celebrity to use to agitate for social change, much of that power and celebrity is drawn from our association with reasoned discourse and its ability to influence democratic processes. So, in our attempt to effect social change, we simultaneously employ and interrogate norms. We use concepts and modes of argument while acknowledging their contingency and what (and who) they exclude. We engage in theory, reasoning, and activism.[28]

Parker appears to argue that Andre stops short at an "engaged bioethics" because she fears going the whole activist route would do violence to the basis of our shared enterprise. We would lose important elements of tentativeness and reflection; we would prematurely cut off discussion; we would give up reason in favor of political muscle (which we probably lack anyway). Parker asserts that bioethics can be activist—indeed, already is activist—and still retain all these desirable qualities.[29]

Of course, we can still screw up. But we don't screw up *because* we have abandoned reason and reflection for activism. Sometimes our mistake will be rushing too quickly to embrace activist methods; other times it will be too much hesitation. The dual nature of our activity can trip us up, but it also represents our strength.[30] To update the classic quotation, we should act as people of thought, and think as people of action.[31]

If we accept this challenge, I see a bright future for the exciting and evolving field of bioethics.

NOTES TO CHAPTER 12

1. One of the standard sources on medical professionalism today is the Medical professionalism project. Medical professionalism in the new millennium: a physicians' charter. *Lancet* 359:520–2, 2002.
2. Stern DT, ed. *Measuring medical professionalism.* New York: Oxford University Press, 2006.
3. An example of an appropriately skeptical view is Hafferty F. Measuring professionalism: a commentary. In: Stern DT, ed. *Measuring medical professionalism.* New York: Oxford University Press, 2006, pp. 281–306.
4. See, for example, Sox HC. The ethical foundations of professionalism: a sociologic history. *Chest* 131:1532–40, 2007.
5. Two important exceptions are Jonsen AR. Watching the doctor. *N Engl J Med* 308:1531–5, 1983; and McCullough LB. The physician's virtues and legitimate self-interest in the patient–physician contract. *Mt Sinai J Med* 60:11–4, 1993.
6. See for example Mariner WK. Business vs. medical ethics: conflicting standards for managed care. *J Law Med Ethics* 23:236–46, 1995; Andre J. The alleged incompatibility of business and medical ethics. *HEC Forum* 11:288–92, 1999.
7. Weber L. *Profits before people? Ethical standards and the marketing of prescription drugs.* Bloomington, IN: Indiana University Press, 2006.
8. For this reason I find it worrisome that Jonathan Moreno devotes a chapter in his survey of bioethics to neuroethics, but barely mentions dementia; Moreno JD. *Is there an ethicist in the house? On the cutting edge of bioethics.* Bloomington, IN: Indiana University Press, 2005, pp. 219–33.
9. For example, Smith WJ. *Culture of death: the assault on medical ethics in America.* San Francisco: Encounter Books, 2001.
10. I am grateful to Julie Kutac for her unpublished survey of extant dementia "pathographies."

11. Campbell EG, Weissman JS, Ehringhaus S, et al. Institutional academic–industry relationships. *JAMA* 298:1779–86, 2007.
12. The book is Brody H. *Hooked: ethics, the medical profession, and the pharmaceutical industry.* Lanham, MD: Rowman and Littlefield, 2007. The blog may be found at www.brodyhooked.blogspot.com.
13. Finucane TE, Christmas C, Travis K. Tube feeding in patients with advanced dementia: a review of the evidence. *JAMA* 282:1365–70, 1999; Winter SM. Terminal nutrition: framing the debate for the withdrawal of nutritional support in terminally ill patients. *Am J Med* 109:723–6, 2000.
14. Klevins RM, Morrison MA, Nadle J, et al. Invasive methicillin-resistant *Staphylococcus aureus* infections in the United States. *JAMA* 2007; 298:1763–71.
15. Thomas D. *The doctor and the devils.* Norfolk, CT: New Directions, 1953. The screenplay is based on the nineteenth-century Edinburgh anatomist Robert Knox's relationship with the murderers Burke and Hare, who supplied him with fresh cadavers, and into whose methods of obtaining their corpses Knox elected not to inquire too closely.
16. Andre J. *Bioethics as practice.* Chapel Hill, NC: University of North Carolina Press, 2002, p. 219.
17. See for example Marshall MF. ASBH and moral tolerance. In: Eckenweiler LA, Cohn FG, eds. *The ethics of bioethics: mapping the moral landscape.* Baltimore: Johns Hopkins University Press, 2007, pp. 134–43.
18. Andre J. *Bioethics as practice*, p. 208. Elsewhere in this volume Andre stresses moral development, more than moral reasoning or moral decision-making, as the core task of bioethics.
19. Andre J. *Bioethics as practice*, p. 219.
20. Andre J. *Bioethics as practice*, p. 221.
21. Parker LS. Bioethics as activism. In: Eckenweiler LA, Cohn FG, eds. *The ethics of bioethics: mapping the moral landscape*, pp. 144–57.
22. Kelly SE. Public bioethics and publics: consensus, boundaries, and participation in biomedical science policy. *Science, Technology & Human Values* 2003; 28:339–64.
23. See for example Moreno JD. Consensus, contracts, and committees. *J Med Philos* 16:393–408, 1991; Moreno JD. *Deciding together: bioethics and moral consensus.* New York: Oxford University Press, 1995.
24. Rawls J. *Political liberalism.* New York: Columbia University Press, 1993.
25. Parker LS. Bioethics as activism. In: Eckenweiler LA, Cohn FG, eds. *The ethics of bioethics: mapping the moral landscape*, pp. 144–57, esp. p. 146.
26. Compare the discussion of the different senses of "race" in Chapter 8.
27. Parker LS. Bioethics as activism. In: Eckenweiler LA, Cohn FG, eds. *The ethics of bioethics: mapping the moral landscape*, p. 151 (citation omitted).
28. Parker LS. Bioethics as activism. In: Eckenweiler LA, Cohn FG, eds. *The ethics of bioethics: mapping the moral landscape*, p. 152.
29. Kayhan Parsi and Karen Geraghty might add here that if we are puzzled in describing precisely what role we expect the bioethicist to play, it is perhaps because we have forgotten the important American tradition of

the public intellectual: Parsi KP, Geraghty KE. The bioethcist as public intellectual. *Am J Bioeth* 4(1):W17–W23, 2004.

30. One should not overstate the extent to which democratic deliberation and activism are compatible. Iris Marion Young argues that often, both are necessary to promote justice; yet they remain in tension; Young IM. Activist challenges to deliberative democracy. *Political Theory* 29:670–90, 2001.

31. *The Columbia World of Quotations*. New York: Columbia University Press, 1996, attributes the original quotation to Ghanaian president Kwame Nkrumah (1900–1972): "...men who think as men of action and act as men of thought" (1964). (Available at: http://www.bartleby.com/66/; accessed September 10, 2008.) I have seen the same basic quotation attributed to Henri Bergson and others.

# Bibliography ⁛

Abrahams E, Ginsburg GS, Silver M. The Personalized Medicine
    Coalition: goals and strategies. *Am J Pharmacogenomics* 5:345–55,
    2005.
Alexander GC, Kurlander J, Wynia MK. Physicians in retainer
    ("concierge") practice. A national survey of physician, patient, and
    practice characteristics. *J Gen Intern Med* 20:1079–83, 2005.
American College of Physicians. *The advanced medical home: a
    patient-centered, physician-guided model of health care.* Philadelphia:
    American College of Physicians, January 30, 2006; http://www.
    acponline.org/hpp/adv_med.pdf (accessed January 30, 2007).
American Medical Association Board of Trustees. Legal interventions
    during pregnancy: court-ordered medical treatments and legal
    penalties for potentially harmful behavior by pregnant women.
    *JAMA* 264:2663–70, 1990.
Andre J. Learning to see: moral growth during medical training. *J Med
    Ethics* 18:148–52, 1992.
Andre J. The alleged incompatibility of business and medical ethics.
    *HEC Forum* 11:288–92, 1999.
Andre J. *Bioethics as practice.* Chapel Hill, NC: University of North
    Carolina Press, 2002.
Angeles J, Somers SA. From policy to action: addressing racial and
    ethnic disparities at the ground-level. Center for Health Care
    Strategies Issue Brief, August 2007, http://www.chcs.org/usr_doc/
    From_Policy_to_Action.pdf (accessed August 25, 2007).

Angell M. The ethics of research in the Third World. *N Engl J Med* 337:847–9, 1997.

Annas GJ. When suicide prevention becomes brutality: the case of Elizabeth Bouvia. *Hastings Cent Rep* 14(2):20–21, 1984.

Annas GJ. Testing poor pregnant women for cocaine—physicians as police investigators. *N Engl J Med* 344:1729–32, 2001.

Anonymous. Complex problems for MDs: as science gains, moral dilemmas intensify. *Am Med News*, May 1, 1972:7.

Anonymous. Navel-gazing: bioethics and the unbearable whiteness of being [editorial]. *New Atlantis* (2):98–100, 2003.

Anonymous. Do researchers learn to practice misbehavior? (letter). *Hastings Cent Rep* 36(2):4, 2006.

Arras J. Nice story, but so what? narrative and justification in ethics. In: Nelson HL, ed. *Stories and their limits: narrative approaches to bioethics*. New York: Routledge, 1997, pp. 65–88.

Asch A. Recognizing death while affirming life: can end of life reform uphold a disabled person's interest in continued life? *Hastings Cent Rep* 35(6):S31–S36, 2005.

Associated Press. Financial ties link docs, drug companies: Minn. Law shines light into money big pharma spends on panel members. MSNBC.com, August 21, 2007; http://www.msnbc.msn.com/id/20379563/ (accessed January 2, 2008).

Auerbach AD, Landefeld CS, Shojania KG. The tension between needing to improve care and knowing how to do it. *N Engl J Med* 357:608–13, 2007.

Baker RB, McCullough LB. Introduction. In: Baker RB, McCullough LB, ed. *Cambridge world history of medical ethics*. New York: Cambridge University Press (in press).

Baldwin J. On being white...and other lies. In: Roediger DR, ed. *Black on white: black writers on what it means to be white*. New York: Schocken Books, 1984.

Balint M. *The doctor, the patient, and his illness*. New York: International Universities Press, 1957.

Banks J, Marmot M, Oldfield Z, et al. Disease and disadvantage in the United States and in England. *JAMA* 295(17):2037–45, 2006.

Banks JT. Literature as a clinical capacity: commentary on "the Quasimodo Complex." *J Clin Ethics* 1:227–31, 1990.

Barnard D. The physician as priest, revisited. *J Religion Health* 24:272–86, 1985.

Barnard D. In the high court of South Africa, case number 4138/98: the global politics of access to low-cost AIDS drugs in poor countries. *Kennedy Inst Ethics J* 12:159–74, 2002.

Baron EM, Denmark FL. An exploration of female genital mutilation. *Ann NY Acad Sci* 1087:339–55, 2006.

Bartlett E. *The history, diagnosis, and treatment of the fevers of the United States.* Philadelphia: Lea and Blanchard, 1847.

Bass MJ, Buck C, Turner L, et al. The physician's actions and the outcome of illness in family practice. *J Fam Pract* 23:43–7, 1986.

Bass BJ, McWhinney IR, Dempsey JB, et al. Predictors of outcomes in headache patients presenting to family physicians—a one year prospective study. *Headache J* 26:285–94, 1986.

Beal AC, Doty MM, Hernandez SE, et al. Closing the divide: how medical homes promote equity in health care: results from the Commonwealth Fund 2006 health care quality survey. Vol. 62 (June 27, 2007); http://www.commonwealthfund.org/publications/publications_show.htm?doc_id=506814& (accessed August 25, 2007).

Beauchamp TL, Childress JF. *Principles of biomedical ethics*, 5th ed. New York: Oxford University Press, 2001.

Benatar SR, Daar AS, Singer PA. Global health ethics: the rationale for mutual caring. *International Affairs* 79:107–38, 2003.

Bhargava PM. The social, moral, ethical, legal, and political implications of today's biological technologies: an Indian point of view. *Biotechnol J* 1: 34–46, 2006.

Bigelow G. Let there be markets: the evangelical roots of economics. *Harper's Magazine* 310(1860), May 2005:33–8.

Bodenheimer T, Berenson RA, Rudolph P. The primary care-specialty income gap: why it matters. *Ann Intern Med* 146:301–6, 2007.

Bodenheimer T, Wagner EH, Grumbach K. Improving primary care for patients with chronic illness. *JAMA* 288:1775–9, 2002.

Bollier J. Investigators: Dr. Jeffrey McLaughlin received more than $600,000 in payments. *Oshkosh* [WI] *Northwestern*, December 2, 2007.

Bond P. Globalization, pharmaceutical pricing, and South African health policy: managing confrontation with U.S. firms and politicians. *Int J Health Serv* 29:765–92, 1999.

Bonham VL, Citrin T, Warshauer-Baker E, et al. *Community based dialogue: engaging communities of color in the U.S. genetics privacy conversation.* (in press)

Booth WC. *The company we keep: an ethics of fiction*. Berkeley: University of California Press; 1988.

Borry P, Schotsman P, Dierickx K. Evidence-based medicine and its role in ethical decision-making. *J Eval Clin Pract* 12:306–11, 2006.

Bosk CL. *Forgive and remember: managing medical failure*. Chicago: University of Chicago Press, 1979.

Bosk CL. *All God's mistakes: genetic counseling in a pediatric hospital*. Chicago: University of Chicago Press, 1992.

Braddy CM, Files JA. Female genital mutilation: cultural awareness and clinical considerations. *J Midwifery Womens Health* 52:158–63, 2007.

Brody H. Genetic engineering: sizing up the arguments in the post–Louise Brown era. In: Teichler-Zallen D, Clements CD, eds. *Science and morality*. Lexington, MA: Lexington Books, 1982:139–53.

Brody H. *Stories of sickness*. New Haven, CT: Yale University Press, 1987.

Brody H. Ethics, technology, and the human genome project. *J Clin Ethics* 2:278–81, 1991.

Brody H. *The healer's power*. New Haven, CT: Yale University Press, 1992.

Brody H. "My story is broken, can you help me fix it?" Medical ethics and the joint construction of narrative. *Lit Med* 13:79–92, 1994.

Brody H. *Stories of sickness*, 2nd ed. New York: Oxford University Press, 2003.

Brody H. A bioethicist offers an apology. *Lansing City Pulse*, October 6, 2004, http://www.lansingcitypulse.com/041006/features/health.asp (accessed December 29, 2007).

Brody H. *Hooked: ethics, the medical profession, and the pharmaceutical industry*. Lanham, MD: Rowman and Littlefield, 2007.

Brody H, Hunt LM. BiDil: assessing a race-based pharmaceutical. *Ann Fam Med* 4:556–60, 2006.

Brody H, Meghani Z, Greenwald K, eds. *Michael Ryan's writings on medical ethics*. Boston: Springer (in press).

Brody H, Miller FG, Bogdan-Lovis E. Evidence-based medicine: watching out for its friends. *Perspect Biol Med* 48:570–84, 2005.

Broyard A. *Intoxicated by my illness*. New York: Clarkson Potter, 1992.

Burchard EG, Ziv E, Coyle N, et al. The importance of race and ethnic background in biomedical research and clinical practice. *N Engl J Med* 348:1170–5, 2003.

Callahan D. The social sciences and the task of bioethics. *Daedalus* 128:275–94, 1999.

Callahan D. Combining hope, hype and hucksterism. *San Diego Union-Tribune*, October 22, 2004, http://www.signonsandiego.com/uniontrib/20041022/news_z1e22callaha.html (accessed November 11, 2007).

Campbell EG, Weissman JS, Ehringhaus S, et al. Institutional academic-industry relationships. *JAMA* 298:1779–86, 2007.

The Cardiac Arrhythmia Suppression Trial (CAST) investigators. Preliminary report: effect of encainide and flecainide on mortality in a randomized trial of arrhythmia suppression after myocardial infarction. *N Engl J Med* 321:406–12, 1989.

Carson RA. Medical ethics as reflective practice. In: Carson RA, Burns CR, ed. *Philosophy of medicine and bioethics*. Boston: Kluwer Academic Publishers, 1997, pp. 181–91.

Carson RA. Focusing on the human scene. Thoughts on problematic theology. In: Davis DS, Zoloth L, eds. *Notes from a narrow ridge: religion and bioethics*. Hagerstown, MD: University Publishing Group, 1999.

Chambers T. *The fiction of bioethics: cases as literary texts*. New York: Routledge, 1999.

Charatan F. US "boutique medicine" could threaten care for the majority. *BMJ* 324:187, 2002.

Charon R. Narrative contributions to medical ethics: recognition, formulation, interpretation, and validation in the practice of the ethicist. In: DuBose ER, Hamel RP, O'Connell LJ, eds. *A matter of principles? Ferment in U.S. bioethics*. Valley Forge, PA: Trinity Press International, 1994, pp. 260–83.

Charon R. *Narrative medicine: honoring the stories of illness*. New York: Oxford University Press, 2006.

Childress JF. Religion, theology and bioethics. In: Miller FG, Fletcher JC, Humber JM, eds. *The nature and prospect of bioethics: interdisciplinary perspectives*. Totowa, NJ: Humana Press, 2003 pp. 43–67.

Clark B. *Whose life is it anyway?* New York: Dodd, Mead, 1979.

Cohen E. Conservative bioethics and the search for wisdom. *Hastings Cent Rep* 36(1):44–56, 2006.

Cohen JJ. Viewpoint: linking professionalism to humanism: what it means, why it matters. *Acad Med* 82:1029–32, 2007.

Conroy AM. Female genital mutilation: whose problem, whose solution? *BMJ* 333:106–7, 2006.

Daly J. *Evidence-based medicine and the search for a science of clinical care*. Berkeley, CA: University of California Press, 2005.

Daniels N. *Just health care.* New York: Cambridge University Press, 1985.

Daniels N. Equity and population health: toward a broader bioethics agenda. *Hastings Cent Rep* 36(4):22–35, 2006.

Davis DS. Rich cases: the ethics of thick description. *Hastings Cent Rep* 21(4):12–17, 1991.

Davis K, Schoen C, Guterman S, et al. *Slowing the growth of U.S. health care expenditures: what are the options?* New York: The Commonwealth Fund, January, 2007:12, 22–23, http://www.cmwf.org/usr_doc/Davis_slowinggrowthUShltcareexpenditureswhatareoptions_989.pdf (accessed February 1, 2007).

Davis K, Schoenbaum SC, Audet AM. A 2020 vision of patient-centered primary care. *J Gen Intern Med* 20:953–57, 2005.

De Vries R. How can we help? From "sociology in" to "sociology of" bioethics. *J Law Med Ethics* 32:279–92, 2004.

De Vries R, Conrad P. Why bioethics needs sociology. In: De Vries R, Subedi J, eds. *Bioethics and society: constructing the ethical enterprise.* Upper Saddle River, NJ: Prentice-Hall, 1998, pp. 233–57.

Doran T, Fullwood C, Gravelle H, et al. Pay-for-performance programs in family practice in the United Kingdom. *N Engl J Med* 355:375–84, 2006.

Doyle AC. *The memoirs of Sherlock Holmes,* ed. C. Roden. New York: Oxford University Press, 1993.

Ehrich K, Williams C, Farsides B, et al. Choosing embryos: ethical complexity and relational autonomy in staff accounts of PGD. *Sociol Health Illn* 29:1091–106, 2007.

Elliott C. Pharma goes to the laundry: public relations and the business of medical education. *Hastings Cent Rep* 34(5):18–23, 2004.

Elliott C. The tyranny of expertise. In: Eckenwiler LA, Cohn FG, eds. *The ethics of bioethics: mapping the moral landscape.* Baltimore: Johns Hopkins University Press, 2007, pp. 43–6.

Emanuel EJ, Wendler D, Killen J, Grady C. What makes clinical research ethical in developing countries ethical? The benchmarks of ethical research. *J Infect Dis* 189:930–37, 2004.

Engel GL. The need for a new medical model: a challenge to biomedicine. *Science* 196:129–36, 1977.

Engel GL. How long must medicine's science be bound by a seventeenth century world view? In: White KL (ed.). *The task of medicine: dialogue at Wickenberg.* Menlo Park, CA: Henry J. Kaiser Family Foundation, 1988, pp. 113–36.

Engelhardt HT Jr. Rights to health care, social justice, and fairness in health care allocations: frustrations in the face of finitude. In: *The foundations of bioethics*, 2nd ed. New York: Oxford University Press, 1996.

Engelhardt HT Jr. Bioethics as politics: a critical reassessment. In: Eckenwiler LA, Cohn FG, eds. *The ethics of bioethics: mapping the moral landscape*. Baltimore: Johns Hopkins University Press, 2007, pp. 118–33.

Epstein AM. Paying for performance in the United States and abroad [editorial]. *N Engl J Med* 355:406–8, 2006.

Evans JH. *Playing God? Human genetic engineering and the rationalization of public bioethical debate*. Chicago: University if Chicago Press, 2002.

Faden RR. Bioethics: a field in transition. *J Law Med Ethics* 2004; 32:276–8.

Farmer P. *Pathologies of power: health, human rights, and the new war on the poor*. Berkeley, CA: University of California Press, 2003.

Farmer P. Campos NG. New malaise: bioethics and human rights in the global era. *J Law Med Ethics* 32:243–51, 2004.

Finucane TE, Christmas C, Travis K. Tube feeding in patients with advanced dementia: a review of the evidence. *JAMA* 282:1365–70, 1999.

Fisher ES, Wennberg DE, Stukel TA, et al. The implications of regional variations in Medicare spending. Part 1: the content, quality, and accessibility of care. *Ann Intern Med* 138:273–87, 2003.

Fisher ES, Wennberg DE, Stukel TA, et al. The implications of regional variations in Medicare spending. Part 2: health outcomes and satisfaction with care. *Ann Intern Med* 138:288–98, 2003.

Fleck LM. Just health care rationing: a democratic decisionmaking approach. *U Penn Law Rev* 140:1597–636, 1992.

Fleck LM. Just caring: Oregon, health care rationing, and informed democratic deliberation. *J Med Philos* 19:367–88, 1994.

Fleck LM. Creating public conversation about behavioral genetics. In: Parens E, Chapman AR, Press N, eds. *Wrestling with behavioral genetics: science, ethics, and public conversation*. Baltimore: The Johns Hopkins Press, 2006, pp. 257–85.

Fletcher F. *Situation ethics: the new morality*. Philadelphia: Westminster Press, 1966.

Fletcher J. *The ethics of genetic control: ending reproductive roulette*. Garden City, NY: Anchor, 1974.

Flexner A. *Medical education in the United States and Canada*. New York: Carnegie Foundation, 1910.

Francis LP, Battin MP, Jacobson JA, Smith CB, et al. How infectious diseases got left out—and what this omission might have meant for bioethics. *Bioethics* 19:307–22, 2005.

Frank A. *The wounded storyteller: body, illness, and ethics*. Chicago: University of Chicago Press, 1995.

Frank AW. *The renewal of generosity: illness, medicine, and how to live*. Chicago: University of Chicago Press, 2004.

Freedman B. Equipoise and the ethics of clinical research. *N Engl J Med* 317:141–5, 1987.

Garcia JLA. Revisiting African American perspectives on biomedical ethics: distinctiveness and other questions. In: Prograis L Jr., Pellegrino ED, eds. *African American bioethics: culture, race, and identity*. Washington, DC: Georgetown University Press, 2007, pp. 1–23.

Garland MJ, Hasnain R. Health care in common: setting priorities in Oregon. *Hastings Cent Rep* 20(5):16–18, 1990.

Gambia Government/Medical Research Council Joint Ethical Committee. Ethical issues facing medical research in developing countries. *Lancet* 351:286–7, 1998.

Geertz C. *The interpretation of cultures*. New York: Basic Books, 1973.

Gillon R. Medical ethics: four principles plus attention to scope. *BMJ* 309:184–8, 1994.

Glickman SW, Ou FS, DeLong ER, et al. Pay for performance, quality of care, and outcomes in acute myocardial infarction. *JAMA* 297:2373–80, 2007.

Goldenberg MJ. On evidence and evidence-based medicine: lessons from the philosophy of science. *Soc Sci Med* 62: 2621–32, 2006.

Goodman KW. *Ethics and evidence-based medicine: fallibility and responsibility in clinical science*. New York: Cambridge University Press, 2003.

GRADE Working Group. Grading quality of evidence and strength of recommendations. *BMJ* 328:1490, 2004.

Green AR, Carney DR, Pallin DJ, et al. Implicit bias among physicians and its prediction of thrombolysis decisions for black and white patients. *J Gen Intern Med* 22:1231–38, 2007.

Greene JA. *Prescribing by numbers: drugs and the definition of disease*. Baltimore: Johns Hopkins University Press, 2007.

Grossman J, MacKenzie FJ. The randomized controlled trial: gold standard, or merely standard? *Perspect Biol Med* 48:517–34, 2005.

Gruenbaum E. Socio-cultural dynamics of female genital cutting: research findings, gaps, and directions. *Cult Health Sex* 7:429–41, 2005.

Guttmacher AE, Collins FS. Genomic medicine–a primer. *N Eng J Med* 347:1512–20, 2002.

Guyatt G, Rennie D, eds. *User's guide to the medical literature: a manual for evidence-based clinical practice.* Chicago: AMA Press, 2002.

Haakonssen L. *Medicine and morals in the Enlightenment: John Gregory, Thomas Percival, and Benjamin Rush.* Atlanta: Rodopi, 1997.

Hafferty F. Measuring professionalism: a commentary. In: Stern DT, ed. *Measuring medical professionalism.* New York: Oxford University Press, 2006, pp. 281–306.

Hahn RA. Division of labor: obstetrician, woman, and society in *Williams Obstetrics*, 1903–1985. *Med Anthropol Q* 1 (new series): 256–82, 1987.

Hahn RA. Why race is differently classified on U.S. birth and infant death certificates: an examination of two hypotheses. *Epidemiol* 10:108–11, 1999.

Hannay DR. *The symptom iceberg: a study of community health.* Boston: Routledge and Kegan Paul, 1979.

Haraway D. Modest witness: feminist diffractions in science studies. In: Galison P, Stump D, eds. *The disunity of science: boundaries, contexts, and power.* Stanford, CA: Stanford University Press, 1996.

Hawkins AH. Literature, medical ethics, and epiphanic knowledge. *J Clin Ethics* 5:283–90, 1994.

Hoffmaster B. What does vulnerability mean? *Hastings Cent Rep* 36(2):38–45, 2006.

Howell JD. *Technology and the hospital: transforming patient care in the early twentieth century.* Baltimore: Johns Hopkins University Press, 1995.

Institute of Medicine. *Coverage matters: insurance and health care.* Washington, DC: National Academy Press; 2001.

Institute of Medicine. *Unequal treatment: confronting racial and ethnic disparities in health care.* Washington, DC: National Academies Press, 2003.

Jackson DZ. Another era of willful white ignorance. *Boston Globe*, July 4, 2007:A9.

Jennings B. A grassroots movement in bioethics. *Hastings Cent Rep* 18(3, suppl) 1–15, 1988.

Jennings B. Possibilities of consensus: toward a democratic moral discourse. *J Med Philos* 16:447–63, 1991.

Jennings B. Traumatic brain injury and the goals of care. The ordeal of reminding. *Hastings Cent Rep* 36(2):29–37, 2006.

Jensen R. *The heart of whiteness: confronting race, racism, and white privilege.* San Francisco: City Lights; 2005.

Johnson H, Broder DS. *The system: the American way of politics at the breaking point.* Boston: Little, Brown, 1996.

Johnson M. *Moral imagination: implications of cognitive science for ethics.* Chicago: University of Chicago Press, 1993.

Jones CP. Invited commentary: "race," racism, and the practice of epidemiology. *Am J Epidemiol* 154: 299–304, 2001.

Jones AH. Narrative based medicine: narrative in medical ethics. *BMJ* 318:253–6, 1999.

Jones JW, McCullough LB, Richman BW. Ethics of boutique medical practice. *J Vasc Surg* 39:1354–5, 2004.

Jonsen AR. Ethics, the law, and the treatment of seriously ill newborns. In: Doudera AE, Peters JD, eds. *Legal and ethical aspects of treating critically and terminally ill patients.* Ann Arbor, MI: AUPHA Press, 1982:236–41.

Jonsen AR. Watching the doctor. *N Engl J Med* 308:1531-5, 1983.

Jonsen AR Beating up bioethics [review essay]. *Hastings Cent Rep* 31(5):40–5, 2001.

Jonsen AR, Toulmin S. *The abuse of casuistry.* Berkeley, CA: University of California Press, 1988.

Kahn J. How a drug becomes "ethnic": law, commerce, and the production of racial categories in medicine. *Yale J Health Policy Law Ethics* 4:1–46, 2004.

Kahn J, Mastroianni A. Introduction: looking forward in bioethics. *J Law Med Ethics* 32:196–97, 2004.

Kane FI. Keeping Elizabeth Bouvia alive for the public good. *Hastings Cent Rep* 15(6):5–8, 1985.

Kaplan SH, Greenfield S, Ware JE. Assessing the effects of physician–patient interactions on the outcome of chronic disease. *Med Care* 27:S110–S127, 1989.

Kass LR. Babies by means of in vitro fertilization: unethical experiments on the unborn? *N Engl J Med* 285:1174–9, 1971.

Kass L[R]. The wisdom of repugnance. *New Republic* 216 (June 2, 1997):17–26.

Kass NE. Public health ethics: from foundations and frameworks to justice and global public health. *J Law Med Ethics* 32:232–42, 2004.

Kassirer JP. Managing care–should we adopt a new ethic? *N Engl J Med* 339:397–8, 1998.

Kassirer JP. *On the take: how medicine's complicity with big business can endanger your health.* New York: Oxford University Press, 2005.

Kelly SE. Public bioethics and publics: consensus, boundaries, and participation in biomedical science policy. *Science, Technology & Human Values* 28:339–64, 2003.

Kelly SE, Marshall PA, Sanders LM, Raffin TA, Koenig BA. Understanding the process of ethics consultation: results of an ethnographic multi-site study. *J Clin Ethics* 8:136–49, 1997.

Kemp S, Squires J, eds. *Feminisms (Oxford readers).* New York: Oxford University Press, 1998.

King P. Race, equity, health policy, and the African American community. In: Prograis L Jr., Pellegrino ED, eds. *African American bioethics: culture, race, and identity.* Washington, DC: Georgetown University Press, 2007, pp. 67–92.

Klevins RM, Morrison MA, Nadle J, et al. Invasive methicillin-resistant *Staphylococcus aureus* infections in the United States. *JAMA* 298:1763–71, 2007.

Klugman CM. The bioethicist: superhero or supervillain? *ASBH Exchange* 10(1):1, 6–7, 2007.

Kuhn TS. *The structure of scientific revolutions.* 2nd ed. Chicago: University of Chicago Press; 1962.

Kopelman LM. The incompatibility of the United Nations' goals and conventionalist ethical relativism. *Developing World Bioethics* 5:234–43, 2005.

Kothari S. Clinical (mis)judgments of quality of life after disability. *J Clin Ethics* 15:300–7, 2004.

Lane SD, Rubenstein RA. Judging the other: responding to traditional female genital surgeries. *Hastings Cent Rep* 26(3):31–40, 1996.

Latham SR. Review of Robert M. Veatch, Disrupted Dialogue: Medical Ethics and the Collapse of Physician-Humanist Dialogue, 1770–1980. *Am J Bioethics* 7:95–96, 2007.

Leake CD. Preface. In: Leake CD, ed. *Percival's medical ethics.* Baltimore: Williams and Wilkins, 1927.

Levenstein JH, McCracken EC, McWhinney IR, et al. The patient-centred clinical method. 1. A model for the doctor-patient interaction in family medicine. *Fam Pract* 3:24–30, 1986.

Levine C. Analyzing Pandora's box: a history of bioethics. In: Eckenwiler LA, Cohn FG, eds. *The ethics of bioethics: mapping the moral landscape.* Baltimore: Johns Hopkins University Press, 2007, pp. 3–23.

Lexchin J, Bero LA, Djulbegovic B, Clark O. Pharmaceutical industry sponsorship and research outcome and quality: systematic review. *BMJ* 326:1167–70, 2003.

Lindemann H. Bioethics' gender. *Am J Bioethics* 6(2):W15–W19, 2006.

Litton P. Nanoethics: what's new? *Hastings Cent Rep* 37(1):22–25, 2007.

Loewy EH. Bioethics: past, present, and an open future. *Camb Q Healthc Ethics* 11:388–97, 2002.

Loughlin M. A platitude too far: "Evidence-based ethics." Commentary on Borry (2006), evidence-based medicine and its role in ethical decision-making. Journal of Evaluation in Clinical Practice 12, 306–311. *J Eval Clin Pract* 12:312–8, 2006.

Lurie P, Wolfe SM. Unethical trials of interventions to reduce perinatal transmission of the human immunodeficiency virus in developing countries. *N Engl J Med* 337:853–56, 1997.

MacIntyre A. *After virtue: a study in moral theory.* Norte Dame, IN: University of Notre Dame Press, 1984.

Macklin R. *Against relativism: cultural diversity and the search for ethical universals in medicine.* New York: Oxford University Press, 1999.

Macklin R. The new conservatives in bioethics: who are they and what do they seek? *Hastings Cent Rep* 36(1):34–43, 2006.

Mariner WK. Business vs. medical ethics: conflicting standards for managed care. *J Law Med Ethics* 23:236–46, 1995.

Marshall MF. ASBH and moral tolerance. In: Eckenweiler LA, Cohn FG, eds. *The ethics of bioethics: mapping the moral landscape.* Baltimore: Johns Hopkins University Press, 2007, pp. 134–43.

Marshall PA. Anthropology and bioethics. *Med Anthropol Q* 6:49–73, 1992.

Marshall P, Koenig B. Accounting for culture in a globalized bioethics. *J Law Med Ethics* 32:252–66, 2004.

Martensen R. Thought styles among the medical humanities: past, present, and near-term future. In: Carson RA, Burns CR, Cole TR, eds. *Practicing the medical humanities: engaging physicians and patients.* Hagerstown, MD: University Publishing Group, 2003, pp. 99–122.

Martin JC, Avant RF, Bowman MA, et al. The future of family medicine: a collaborative project of the family medicine community. *Ann Fam Med* 2 (Suppl 1): S3–S32, 2004.

Martone M. Traumatic brain injury and the goals of care. *Hastings Cent Rep* 36(2):3, 2006.

May WF. *The patient's ordeal*. Bloomington, IN: Indiana University Press, 1991.

McCullough LB. The physician's virtues and legitimate self-interest in the patient-physician contract. *Mt Sinai J Med* 60:11–14, 1993.

McCullough LB, ed. *John Gregory and the invention of professional medical ethics and the profession of medicine*. Boston: Kluwer Academic Publishers, 1998.

Medical professionalism project. Medical professionalism in the new millennium: a physicians' charter. *Lancet* 359:520-2, 2002.

Miles A, Polychronis A, Grey JE. The evidence-based health care debate–2006. Where are we now? [editorial introduction and commentary]. *J Eval Clin Pract* 12:239–47, 2006.

Miller BL. Autonomy and the refusal of lifesaving treatment. *Hastings Cent Rep* 11(4):22–8, 1981.

Miller FG. Revisiting the Belmont Report: the ethical significance of the distinction between clinical research and medical care. *APA Newsletter on Philosophy and Medicine* 5(2):10–14, 2005.

Miller FG, Fletcher JC, Humber JM, eds. *The nature and prospect of bioethics: interdisciplinary perspectives*. Totowa, NJ: Humana Press, 2003.

Miller FG, Brody H. A critique of clinical equipoise. Therapeutic misconception in the ethics of clinical trials. *Hastings Cent Rep* 33(3):19–28, 2003.

Mondale WF. The issues before us. *Hastings Cent Rep* 1(1):1, June 1971.

Montgomery K. Medical ethics: literature, literary studies, and the question of interdisciplinarity. In: Miller FG, Fletcher JC, Humber JM, ed. *The nature and prospect of bioethics: interdisciplinary perspectives*. Totowa, NJ: Humana Press, 2003, pp. 141–78.

Montgomery K. *How doctors think: clinical judgment and the practice of medicine*. New York: Oxford University Press, 2006.

Moreno JD. Consensus, contracts, and committees. *J Med Philos* 16:393–408, 1991.

Moreno JD. *Deciding together: bioethics and moral consensus*. New York: Oxford University Press, 1995.

Moreno JD. Goodbye to all that: the end of moderate protectionism in human subjects research. *Hastings Cent Rep* 31(3):9–17, 2001.

Moreno JD. In the wake of Katrina: has "bioethics" failed? *Am J Bioethics* 5(5): W18–W19, 2005.

Moreno JD. *Is there an ethicist in the house? On the cutting edge of bioethics.* Bloomington, IN: Indiana University Press, 2005.

Morreim EH. At the intersection of medicine, law, economics, and ethics: bioethics and the art of intellectual cross-dressing. In: Carson RA, Burns CR, eds. *Philosophy of medicine and bioethics.* Boston: Kluwer Academic Publishers, 1997:299–325.

Morrison I. *Health care in the new millenium: visions, values, and leadership.* San Francisco: Jossey-Bass, 2000.

Murray CJ, Kulkarni SC, Michaud C, et al. Eight Americas: investigating mortality disparities across races, counties, and race-counties in the United States. *PLoS Med* 3(9), 2006 [epub].

Murray TH. Even if it worked, cloning wouldn't bring her back. *Washington Post,* April 8, 2001:B1.

Murray TH, Jennings B. The quest to reform end-of-life care: rethinking assumptions and setting new directions. *Hastings Cent Rep* 35(6 suppl):S52–S57, 2005.

Mykhalovskiy E, Weir L. The problem of evidence-based medicine: directions for social science. *Soc Sci Med* 59:1059–69, 2004.

Myser C. Differences from somewhere: the normativity of whiteness in bioethics in the United States. *Am J Bioethics* 3(2):1–11, 2003.

Myser C. Community-based participatory research in United States bioethics: steps toward more democratic theory and policy. *Am J Bioethics* 4:67–68, 2004.

National Bioethics Advisory Commission. *Ethical and policy issues in research involving human participants.* Washington, DC: National Bioethics Advisory Commission, 2001; http://www.bioethics.gov/reports/past_commissions/nbac_human_part.pdf

Nelson HL, ed. *Stories and their limits: narrative approaches to bioethics.* New York: Routledge, 1997.

Nelson HL. Feminist bioethics: where we've been, where we're going. *Metaphilosophy* 31:492–508, 2000.

Nelson HL. *Damaged identities, narrative repair.* Ithaca, NY: Cornell University Press, 2001.

Nussbaum MC. *Frontiers of justice: disability, nationality, species membership.* Cambridge, MA: Belknap/Harvard University Press, 2006, pp. 255–62.

Oberlander J. Health reform interrupted: the unraveling of the Oregon Health Plan. *Health Aff* 26(1):w96–w105, 2006.

Okie S. Teaching hospitals how to listen: one woman struggled to convince administrators that staff responsiveness—or lack of it—affects patient outcomes. *Washington Post,* December 12, 2006:HE1.

Oshinsky DM. *Polio: An American story.* New York: Oxford University Press, 2006.

Parker LS. Bioethics as activism. In: Eckenweiler LA, Cohn FG, eds. *The ethics of bioethics: Mapping the moral landscape.* Baltimore: Johns Hopkins University Press, 2007:144–57.

Parsi KP, Geraghty KE. The bioethicist as public intellectual. *Am J Bioethics* 4(1): W17–W23, 2004.

Pendleton D, Schofield T, Tate P, Havelock P. *The consultation: an approach to learning and teaching.* Oxford: Oxford University Press, 1984.

Percival T. *Medical ethics; or, a code of institutes and precepts adapted to the professional conduct of physicians and surgeons* ... Manchester: Russell, 1803; modern reprint by the Classics of Medicine Library, Birmingham, AL, 1985.

Pellegrino ED. Bioethics as an interdisciplinary enterprise: where does ethics fit in the mosaic of disciplines? In: Carson RA, Burns CR, eds. *Philosophy of medicine and bioethics.* Boston: Kluwer Academic Publishers, 1997:1–23.

Phillips WR. Questioning the Future of Family Medicine. Fam Med 36:664–5, 2004.

Pitts L. Replying to those e-mails about Vick. *Miami Herald,* August 12, 2007, http://www.miamiherald.com/living/columnists/leonard_pitts/story/199338.html (accessed August 24, 2007).

Potter VR. Bioethics: the science of survival. *Perspect Biol Med* 14:127–53, 1970.

Potter VR. *Bioethics: bridge to the future.* Englewood Cliffs, NJ: Prentice-Hall, 1971.

Potter VR. *Global bioethics: building on the Leopold legacy.* East Lansing, MI: Michigan State University Press, 1988.

Porter E. The divisions that tighten the purse strings. *New York Times,* April 29, 2007: Sect. 3, p. 4.

President's Council on Bioethics. *Taking care: ethical care-giving in our aging society.* Washington, DC: President's Council on Bioethics, 2005; http://www.bioethics.gov/reports/taking_care/taking_care.pdf

Pruyser PW. *A dynamic psychology of religion.* New York: Harper and Row, 1968.

Rachels J. When philosophers shoot from the hip: a report from America. *Bioethics* 5(1):67–71, 1991.

Radey C. *Choosing wisely: how patients and their families can make the right decisions about life and death.* New York: Doubleday/Image, 1992.

Ramsey P. Shall we "reproduce"? I. The medical ethics of in vitro fertilization. *JAMA* 220:1346–50, 1972.

Ramsey P. Shall we "reproduce"? II. Rejoinders and future forecast. *JAMA* 220:1480–85, 1972.

Rawls J. *A theory of justice.* Cambridge, MA: Belknap-Harvard University Press, 1971.

Rawls J. *Political liberalism.* New York: Columbia University Press, 1993.

Rawls J. *The law of peoples; with "the idea of public reason" revisited.* Cambridge, MA: Harvard University Press, 1999.

Rawls J. *Justice as fairness: a restatement.* Cambridge, MA: Belknap Press of Harvard University Press, 2001.

Reich WT (ed.) *Encyclopedia of bioethics* (4 vol.) New York: Free Press, 1978.

Reich WT. The word "bioethics": its birth and the legacies of those who shaped it. *Kennedy Inst Ethics J* 4:319–35, 1994.

Reich WT. The word "bioethics": the struggle over its earliest meanings. *Kennedy Inst Ethics J* 5:19–34, 1995.

Reiser SJ. *Medicine and the reign of technology.* New York: Cambridge University Press, 1978.

Rhodes R, Cohen D, Friedman E, et al. Professionalism in medical education. *Am J Bioethics* 4(2):20–2, 2004.

Risch N, Burchard E, Ziv E, et al. Categorization of humans in biomedical research: genes, race and disease. *Genome Biol* 3(7):comment 2007 [epub], 2002.

Rogers C. *Client-centered therapy: its current practice implications and theory.* Cambridge, MA: Riverside, 1951.

Rorty R. Pragmatism, relativism, and irrationalism. In: *Consequences of pragmatism.* Minneapolis: University of Minnesota Press, 1982, pp. 160–75.

Rosenberg CE. The therapeutic revolution: medicine, meaning, and social change in nineteenth century America. In: Vogel MJ, Rosenberg CE, eds. *The therapeutic revolution: essays in the social history of American medicine.* Philadelphia: University of Pennsylvania Press, 1979, pp. 3–25.

Rosenblatt LM. *Literature as exploration.* New York: Modern Language Association, 1995.

Rosenthal MB, Frank RG, Li Z, et al. Early experience with pay-for-performance: from concept to practice. *JAMA* 294:1788–93, 2005

Rothman DJ. *Strangers at the bedside: a history of how law and bioethics transformed medical decision making.* New York: Basic Books, 1991.

Rubin SB, Zoloth L. Clinical ethics and the road less taken: mapping the future by tracking the past. *J Law Med Ethics* 32:218–25, 2004.

Ryan M. *Manual of medical jurisprudence,* 2nd ed. London: Sherwood, Gilbert and Piper, 1836.

Sankar P. Cho MK, Condit CM, et al. Genetic research and health disparities. *JAMA* 291:2985–9, 2004.

Sass HM. Fritz Jahr's 1927 concept of bioethics. *Kennedy Inst Ethics J* 17:279–95, 2007.

Schatz GS. Are the rationale and regulatory system for protecting human subjects of biomedical and behavioral research obsolete and unworkable, or ethically important but inconvenient and inadequately enforced? *J Contemp Health Law Policy* 20:1–31, 2003.

Schneider CE. Hard cases and the politics of righteousness. *Hastings Cent Rep* 35(3):24–7, 2005.

Schwartz RS. Racial profiling in medical research. *N Engl J Med* 344:1392–3, 2001.

Selgelid MJ. Ethics and infectious disease. *Bioethics* 19:272–89, 2005.

Sen A. *Development as freedom.* New York, Anchor Books, 2000.

Sherwin S. *No longer patient: feminist ethics and health care.* Philadelphia: Temple University Press, 1992.

Sia C, Tonniges TF, Osterhus E, et al. History of the medical home concept. *Pediatrics* 113 (5 suppl):1473–8, 2004.

Siegler M. Searching for moral certainty in medicine: a proposal for a new model of the doctor–patient encounter. *Bull NY Acad Med* 57:56–69, 1981.

Smith WJ. *Culture of death: the assault on medical ethics in America.* San Francisco: Encounter Books, 2001.

Snyder L, Neubauer RL. Pay-for-performance principles that promote patient-centered care: an ethics manifesto. *Ann Intern Med* 147:792–94, 2007.

Sox HC. The ethical foundations of professionalism: a sociologic history. *Chest* 131:1532–40, 2007.

Spann SJ, Task Force 6 and the Executive Editorial Team. Report on financing the new model of family medicine. *Ann Fam Med* 2(suppl 3):S1–S21, 2004.

Speth JG. *Red sky at morning: America and the crisis of the global environment.* New Haven, CT: Yale University Press, 2005.

Starfield B, Wray C, Hess K, et al. The influence of patient-practitioner agreement on outcome of care. *Am J Publ Health* 71:127–32, 1981.

Steinbock B, ed. *The Oxford handbook of bioethics*. New York: Oxford University Press, 2007.

Stern DT, ed. *Measuring medical professionalism*. New York: Oxford University Press; 2006.

Stevens MLT. *Bioethics in America: origins and cultural politics*. Baltimore: Johns Hopkins University Press, 2000.

Stevens MLT. History and bioethics. In: Miller FG, Fletcher JC, Humber JM, ed. *The nature and prospect of bioethics: interdisciplinary perspectives*. Totowa, NJ: Humana Press, 2003, pp. 179–96.

Stevens MLT. Intellectual capital and voting booth bioethics: a contemporary historical critique. In: Eckenwiler LA, Cohn FG, eds. *The ethics of bioethics: mapping the moral landscape*. Baltimore: Johns Hopkins University Press, 2007, pp. 59–73.

Stewart M, Brown JB, Weston WW, et al. *Patient-centered medicine: transforming the clinical method*. Thousand Oaks, CA: Sage Publications, 1995.

Striebig BA, Jantzen T, Rowden K. Ethical considerations of the short-term and long-term health impacts, costs, and educational value of sustainable development projects. *Sci Eng Ethics* 12:345–54, 2006.

Tangwa GB. The traditional African perception of a person. Some implications for bioethics. *Hastings Cent Rep* 30(5):39–43, 2000.

Thomas D. *The doctor and the devils*. Norfolk, CT: New Directions, 1953.

Thomas L. The technology of medicine. *N Engl J Med* 285:1366–8, 1971.

Thomas L. *The lives of a cell: notes of a biology-watcher*. New York: Bantam Books, 1975.

Todd KH, Deaton C, D'Adamo AP, Goe L. Ethnicity and analgesic practice. *Ann Emerg Med* 35: 11–6, 2000.

Todd KH, Samaroo N, Hoffman JR. Ethnicity as a risk factor for inadequate emergency department analgesia. *JAMA* 269:1537–39, 1993.

Tonelli MR. Integrating evidence into clinical practice: an alternative to evidence-based approaches. *J Eval Clin Pract* 12:248–56, 2006.

Tresolini CP, Pew-Fetzer Task Force. *Health professions education and relationship-centered care*. San Francisco, CA: Pew Health Professions Commission, 1994.

Trotter G. Left bias in academic bioethics: three dogmas. In: Eckenwiler LA, Cohn FG, eds. *The ethics of bioethics: mapping the moral landscape.* Baltimore: Johns Hopkins University Press, 2007:108–17.

Turner L. Bioethics in a multicultural world: medicine and morality in pluralistic settings. *Health Care Analysis* 11:99–117, 2003.

Tyson J. Evidence-based ethics and the care of premature infants. *Future Child* 5: 197–213, 1995.

Tyson JE, Stoll BJ. Evidence-based ethics and the care and outcome of extremely premature infants. *Clin Perinatol* 30:363–87, 2003.

United States National Bioethics Advisory Commission. *Ethical and policy issues in research involving human participants.* Bethesda, MD: National Bioethics Advisory Commission, 2001.

United States President's Commission for the Study of Ethical Problems in Medicine and Biomedical and Behavioral Research. *Deciding to forego life-sustaining treatment.* Washington, DC: U.S. Government Printing Office, 1983.

Vanderpool HY, ed. *The ethics of research involving human subjects: facing the 21st century.* Frederick, MD: University Publishing Group; 1996.

Veatch RM. *Case studies in medical ethics.* Cambridge, MA: Harvard University Press, 1977.

Veatch RM. Professional ethics: new principles for physicians. *Hastings Cent Rep* 10(3):16–19, 1980.

Veatch RM. *Death, dying and the biological revolution: our last quest for responsibility.* New Haven, CT: Yale University Press, 1989.

Veatch RM. *Disrupted dialogue: medical ethics and the collapse of physician-humanist communication (1770–1980).* New York: Oxford University Press, 2005.

Veatch RM, Gaylin W, Morgan C, eds. *The teaching of medical ethics.* Hastings-on-Hudson, NY: The Hastings Center; 1973.

Vinten-Johansen P, Brody H, Paneth N, et al. *Cholera, chloroform, and the science of medicine: A life of John Snow.* New York: Oxford University Press, 2003.

Walker A. Strong horse tea. In: Secundy MG, Nixon LL, eds. *Trials, tribulations, and celebrations: African-American perspectives on health, illness, aging and loss.* Yarmouth, ME: Intercultural Press, 1992, pp. 76–82.

Walker MU. Keeping moral space open: new images of ethics consulting. *Hastings Cent Rep* 23(2):33–40, 1993.

Walker MU. *Moral understandings: a feminist study in ethics.* New York: Routledge, 1998.

Warner JH. *The therapeutic perspective: medical practice, knowledge, and identity in America, 1820–1885*. Cambridge, MA: Harvard University Press, 1986.

Weber L. *Profits before people? Ethical standards and the marketing of prescription drugs*. Bloomington, IN: Indiana University Press, 2006.

Welch W. Report: 82M went uninsured. *USA Today*, June 15, 2004.

Werner RM, Bradlow ET. Relationship between Medicare's hospital compare performance measures and mortality rates. *JAMA* 296:2694–2702, 2006.

Whitehouse PJ. The rebirth of bioethics: extending the original formulations of Van Rensselaer Potter. *Am J Bioethics* 3(4):W26–W31, 2003.

Wikler D. Presidential address: bioethics and social responsibility. *Bioethics* 11:185–92, 1997.

Williams C. Dilemmas in fetal medicine: premature applications of technology or responding to women's choice? *Sociol Health Illn* 28:1–20, 2006.

Winslade WJ. Intellectual cross-dressing: an eccentricity or a practical necessity? Commentary on Morreim. In: Carson RA, Burns CR, eds. *Philosophy of medicine and bioethics*. Boston: Kluwer Academic Publishers, 1997, pp. 327–34.

Winter SM. Terminal nutrition: framing the debate for the withdrawal of nutritional support in terminally ill patients. *Am J Med* 109:723–6, 2000.

Wisdom J. *Paradox and certainty*. Oxford: Blackwell, 1965.

World Health Organization. *The World Health Report 2000: health systems: improving performance*. Geneva: World Health Organization; 2000.

Young IM. Activist challenges to deliberative democracy. *Political Theory* 29:670–90, 2001.

Zoloth L. I want you: notes toward a theory of hospitality. In: Eckenwiler LA, Cohn FG, eds. *The ethics of bioethics: mapping the moral landscape*. Baltimore: Johns Hopkins University Press, 2007, pp. 205–19.

Zuger A, Miles SH. Physicians, AIDS, and occupational risk: historical traditions and ethical obligations. *JAMA* 258:1924–8, 1987.

# INDEX ⠶

Post-modernism, 118, 142, 225
Potter, Van Renssalaer, 7t, 48n72,
    178–179, 189n2, 189n4, 189n5,
    190n8
Poverty, 182, 205
    See also Globalization and global
    development
Power, 10–11, 16–17, 33, 35–36, 39–40,
    67–70, 73–74, 82, 105–116, 159,
    176n23, 177, 191n22, 206–209, 217,
    224–225, 227–228
Practice, of bioethics, 5, 17, 220, 222
Pragmatism, 6, 121–122, 148
Preprinted forms, as technology,
    197–198
President's Commission on Ethical
    Problems in Medicine, 159, 181
President's Council on Bioethics, 10, 22,
    214n20
Primary care, 7t, 17, 51, 66, 82, 87n49, 99,
    102, 113
    See also Family medicine
Principles and principlism, 23–24, 34,
    114, 119–122, 212n1
Professionalism, 3, 28, 79–81, 86n45, 218,
    220, 229n1
Prophetic role, 33, 45n48, 204
Protease inhibitor drugs, 128
Prudential Foundation, 90
Pruyser, Paul, 34
Public health, ethics of, 7t, 15, 179, 180,
    188, 190n13, 192n27, 205, 209–211
Public intellectual, 230–231n29
PubMed, 65

Quadriplegia, 158
Quality of health care, 154

Race, 4, 7t, 10, 11, 16, 17, 30, 100, 109–110,
    112, 114, 127, 135–157, 228
    Geographic, 140–141
    Senses of, 139–141, 149
    As social construction, 140–141
Rachels, James, 200, 201
Racial Privacy Initiative, 155n9
Racism, 106, 135–136, 147
Ramsey, Paul, 31, 34
Randomized controlled trials, 65, 69,
    72–74, 84n16
Rational democratic deliberation model,
    94, 96t
Rationing of health care, 90–91, 175n20

Rawls, John, 98, 162–164, 175n21, 183,
    190n16, 191n17, 192n31, 226
Reductionism, 38, 51, 53, 57
Reflective equilibrium, 98
Reiser, Stanley, 212–213n6
Relationship-centered care, 52–53
Relativism, 121–124, 131n7, 155n3, 182
Religion, 7t, 22, 26, 31–35, 45n44, 137, 201,
    204, 214n18, 215n28
Reproduction, ethics of, 7t, 112,
    198–200, 207
Research ethics, 5, 7t, 11–14, 20n32, 223
    International, 117, 126–130, 182
    See also Ethics committees, research
    (IRBs)
Resource allocation, 22, 167, 168,
    169–173
Respirator, see Ventilator, mechanical
Revolutionary science, 8, 16
"Right to die," see End-of-life care
Right to health care, 155n1
Right-to-life advocates, 226, 227
Right to vote, 165–166, 174n12
Rights, human, 185, 191n23
Riverside, California, 175n19
Rivlin, David, 158, 169, 170
Robert Wood Johnson Foundation, 90
Rogers, Carl, 52
Rorty, Richard, 121–122
Rosenberg, Charles, 30
Rosenblatt, Louise, 42n19
Rothman, David, 27
Rubenstein, Robert, 126
Rwanda, 124, 187
Ryan, Michael, 26

Sabin polio vaccine, 67–68
Salk polio vaccine, 67–68
San Diego, California, 220
Sanctity of life, 168
Sarah, 59
SARS (severe acute respiratory
    syndrome), 26, 182
Sass, Hans-Martin, 189n2
Schatz, Gerald, 13–14, 20n32
Scheper-Hughes, Nancy, 221–222
Scherger, Joseph, 63n23
Schiavo, Terri, 9, 89, 102n2, 175n17, 180
Scotland, 28, 195, 230n15
Scottish Enlightenment, 28
Self-interest, of physician, 218
Selgelid, Michael, 45n44

Ventilator, mechanical, 27, 51, 67, 88, 158, 169
Vick, Michael, 143
Victorian era, 107–108, 110
Virtue ethics, 31, 218

Walker, Alice, 30
Walker, Margaret Urban, 36, 46n63, 112–114, 122
Warner, John Harley, 213n11
Washington, 90, 211
Washington, D.C., 178, 221
Wasserman, David, 175n16
Weber, Leonard, 219
White privilege, 109, 141–145
Whitehouse, Peter, 179, 190n5

Whiteness, *see* White privilege
Williams, Clare, 206–208, 209, 216n39
Willowbrook study, 12
Winslade, William, 19n18, 41n9
Wisconsin, 178
World Health Organization (WHO), 125, 126, 132n12, 132n17, 174n5
    Ranking of U.S. health system, 14

X-rays, 197–198

Yellow fever, 194
Yeshiva University, 175n16
Young, Iris Marion, 231n30

Zoloth, Laurie, 59